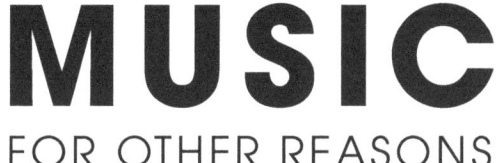

Conversations with Music Therapists

MUSIC
FOR OTHER REASONS

Bob Cowin

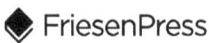
FriesenPress

One Printers Way
Altona, MB R0G 0B0
Canada

www.friesenpress.com

Copyright © 2021 by Bob Cowin
First Edition — 2021

Excerpts used with permission from the following works:

Musicophilia: Tales of Music and the Brain, Book by Oliver Sacks
First Vintage Books edition, 2008
Penguin Random House

Adult with Autism Shines in Music Therapy
Video posted by Ryan Judd
The Rhythm Tree
Exeter, NH

How Music Therapy Changed My Life
Video posted by Children's Hospital Colorado, Aurora, CO

Music Therapy & Emotions for Depression, Stress & Mental Health Issues
Video posted by Hope E. Young
Center for Music Therapy
Austin, TX

My Journey to Music Therapy: Becoming an MT-BC
My Internship Experience: Becoming a Music Therapist
Videos posted by Mai Abe
Creative Vibes Music Therapy
San Jose, CA

Parkinson's and Music Therapy
Video posted by Norton Healthcare
Louisville, KY

Using Music Therapy to Treat Trauma
Video posted by Kelly Meashey
Philadelphia, PA

All rights reserved.

No part of this publication may be reproduced in any form, or by any means, electronic or mechanical, including photocopying, recording, or any information browsing, storage, or retrieval system, without permission in writing from FriesenPress.

ISBN
978-1-03-912829-3 (Hardcover)
978-1-03-912828-6 (Paperback)
978-1-03-912830-9 (eBook)

1. Health & Fitness, Healing

Distributed to the trade by
The Ingram Book Company

For Beth

This is a work of creative non-fiction. Although I've changed many names, taken liberties with details, and occasionally invented dialogue, I've nevertheless portrayed everything that matters as faithfully as possible.

Contents

Setting the Stage

CURIOSITY	3
ONLINE GLIMPSES	11
NEUROSCIENCE	23
BECOMING A THERAPIST	35
SNIPPETS FROM LAYPEOPLE	47

Conversations

ANNETTE	59
ANTONIO	93
MEGAN	115

References	141

Music therapy, to me, is music performance without the ego.
It's not about entertainment as much as it's about empathizing.
If you can use music to slip past the pain
and gather insight into the workings of someone else's mind,
you can begin to fix a problem.

—*Jodi Picoult*

Setting the Stage

CURIOSITY

Amy's impulse had been to decline the invitation from the hospice society. "An hour of making polite conversation with strangers," she explained to me, "could be deadly—no pun intended—even though I'm sure they're all very nice people." She'd never see them again, and their only commonality was having made a donation.

"So the reception was some sort of thank-you tea for donors?" I asked.

"Yes. I was interested in what the staff might say about their work, but I dreaded the mingling before and after the formal program."

In the end, the venue had caused her to relent. "I hadn't been in the university faculty club for years, and I was curious to see what had happened to it. I wondered whether it was still a going concern or if it had become just a lovely west coast space that gets rented out."

"West coast space?"

"Low building of cedar and glass. Blends into the landscape, with lots of earth tones inside."

"Gotcha. I know that style of architecture."

Amy had attended the event, survived the chitchat, and been intrigued by one of the presentations. When I asked what had piqued her interest, she replied that the speaker was a music therapist. "Pleasant lady. Middle-aged and ordinary appearing, but she had an engaging presence. Open and accepting is the best I can describe her. I couldn't tell if this was her natural persona or if she had cultivated it in her profession." Then the speaker had pulled out her Omnichord and Amy was hooked.

I'd never heard of an Omnichord. Amy depicted it merely as a small electronic instrument that I should look up on YouTube. "The cool thing about it," she said, "is that once you push the button for a particular chord, the instrument ensures every note you play with your other hand will harmonize with that chord. Anybody can make some pleasing sounds, adding drum beats and special effects if they feel like it."

The therapist—I think Amy said her name was Janet, though it might have been Jamie—had been employed part-time by the hospice a decade earlier, a member of their pain management and spiritual care teams for the dying. Then the funding for her position had dried up. Only now was the society managing to bring her back on staff, and hence the unspoken request to donors to keep the money flowing.

"I'd never thought of music as important in end-of-life care," Amy mused. "Pleasant background ambience, yes. A distraction or entertainment, yes. But it never occurred to me that music could be used intentionally, say as a catalyst for some deeply meaningful conversations or to pull an Alzheimer's patient temporarily back into this world. Or that a music therapist might be as interested in getting her client to make music as to listen to it. Audience participation, as it were."

"Like singing together? I'd suck at that."

"I don't know, but here's the example she gave. She learned that one of a client's favourite songs was "The Impossible Dream" from some Broadway musical. As he recounted the highlights of his life, she rewrote the lyrics to make them about him. This tickled his fancy, especially as he recalled cherished family vacations, and she made a recording so that he could listen to it after she left.

"At his funeral, that was the song his family played. Maybe for her client it started out as just a little ditty, a diversion. But within minutes it had evolved into something much more meaningful to him. And for his kids it was a profound memory that will stay with them for the rest of their days. How often do we get to touch people that deeply?"

I felt a lump in my throat, but didn't let on. I recounted, "Many years ago, I attended a conference in Seattle where the social event one evening was an hour's train ride to a leisurely dinner in a vineyard. On the return trip, one of the people in our cluster of face-to-face seats was a statistician who had been involved with music therapy in his previous life."

Amy encouraged me with subtle nods while I collected my thoughts.

"He got talking about playing the harp for people who were dying," I said. "I mean, literally at the end. They could be gone in a matter of hours.

"Often breathing patterns change just before death. Maybe you've heard of the death rattle? Whether or not these changes bother the client, they can be hard for their loved ones to observe. My colleague claimed that he could frequently find either the notes or a rhythm that resonated with the breathing, helping it become less laboured and more regular. And the harp was apparently better for this purpose than other types of instruments."

Amy asked, "How significant was that?"

"I can't recall what more he said. It was a long time ago. But what struck me, and what I've remembered all these years, was that he took it for granted that music can, and should, be part of the dying process. It should be therapeutic, not just cosmetic or superficial."

The two of us sat quietly. I'm not very musical, and I usually prefer silence to background music when I'm home alone. Yet even I can get caught up in a bouncy tune or be transported by a haunting melody in a minor key. "I wonder what hidden parts of my being a therapist might be able to reveal through music," I finally said.

Amy chose not to use this opening to make a wisecrack—the topic had also put her in a reflective mood. I never did find out what she was thinking, but all sorts of questions were forming in my mind. I decided to do a little poking about on the Internet because I knew music therapists show up in a wide range of settings, and use a variety of techniques. I just didn't know exactly where and what they did.

As I drove home, I ruminated on how our awareness of music's healing power is hardly new. Three thousand years ago, the Old Testament described music soothing a tormented King Saul. Back in my study, I searched online for "Saul & Harp." I eventually stumbled upon a verse from 1st Samuel: "And whenever the evil spirit from God was upon Saul, David took the lyre and played it with his hand; so Saul was refreshed, and was well, and the evil spirit departed from him."

Nonetheless, I learned from other websites that it took until the 1940s for American universities to begin offering degrees in music therapy. That is, music for health and educational purposes rather than to train performers and composers. During this period, several music organizations began looking into music as a form of treatment, with regional music therapy conferences emerging during World War II. By 1950, a national organization had formed in the USA.

Soldiers hospitalized with combat fatigue and shell shock, ailments now described as types of post-traumatic stress injury, served as the catalyst for these initiatives. Many veterans responded well when a few hospitals hired musicians to play for them, but why the music was helping, and therefore strategies for replicating those successes, remained murky. The musicians realized they needed more training, not as musicians but as therapists.

The Canadian story is even more recent. A landmark conference, attended by only five dozen people, convened at a psychiatric hospital in St. Thomas, Ontario, in the summer of 1974. Over the next couple of years a national group, initially named the Canadian Music Therapy Association, was formed. The first of Canada's six training programs opened in North Vancouver just two years later, and this prompted me to look up the current version of that music therapy program at Capilano University.

Given that certification as a music therapist in Canada or the United States requires a bachelor's degree, I was hardly surprised to learn that Capilano offers a four-and-a-half-year program. Students take prerequisite courses in music, psychology, and other subjects during their first two years of study, and then apply to enter the music therapy program in third year. The application process includes an interview and audition, each critical.

The interview is courteously intimate and has little to do with music. Rather, its purpose is to determine whether the applicant is socially competent and self-aware and fits the program emotionally. The personal attributes the program values in its students, over and above musical ability, are numerous and daunting.

The instructors are not interested in dully conventional applicants, striving instead to attract what they describe as open-minded, spontaneous, and creative individuals. However, neither do they want free spirits who are oblivious to others. They look for musicians who are balanced and flexible, and who show evidence of having internalized holistic and multicultural perspectives. Finally, the screening seeks those who are passionate about self-exploration, eager to nurture their own growth and transformation through lifelong learning, and who exhibit "a good deal of heart."

During the interview, two instructors probe about the applicant's life, their family of origin, and any challenges they may have faced. "The faculty are aware," the website cautions, "that talking about, or showing, emotion is unfamiliar to some people and some cultural backgrounds. The questions in the interview will be sensitive to your background, but please know that the elements of emotion and self-disclosure are important parts of being a music therapist, from our perspective." Perhaps a box of tissues is discreetly placed somewhere in the interview room.

The audition assesses basic competence across the most common tools of the trade: voice, guitar, and piano. Then applicants are asked to perform "two pieces of music that offer contrasting emotions on their main instrument, demonstrating technique and expressiveness." The final component of the audition concerns ear training: singing unaccompanied on key, finding the starting note for a song, hearing the differences among types of chords, and a few other tasks that would thoroughly flummox me. Because therapists are expected to improvise and navigate the music of many eras and cultures, my impression is that a broad musicality is more important than a polished technique in a particular genre.

The Capilano website mentioned a pamphlet from the Canadian Association of Music Therapists, *Music Therapy: A Health Care Profession*. This organization struck me as a good destination for my next stop on the web.

Some pages on the association's website are official and bureaucratic, but I perked up at a section listing typical area of practice. Geriatrics, palliative care, and therapy for the emotionally traumatized I already knew about, while fields such as oncology and obstetrics, where pain and anxiety are issues, immediately made sense to me. I could guess how music might help in the rehabilitation of a brain injury, was vaguer how it would be used with hearing, speech, and vision impairments, but really had no idea how a therapist might work with those on the autism spectrum or with a developmental disability. Evidently, music therapy is part of the toolkit for dealing with substance abuse, risky teenage behaviour, and some mental illnesses.

Rather than assuage my curiosity, my tiny bit of research fanned it. Now I wanted to meet some practitioners to learn what they do, why they do it, and how well it goes. And then I received an email that prompted this project. It was a broadcast message from my acquaintance Jessica about a new volunteer activity for her singing group of five women. "We are now offering our unique gift of *a cappella*, and occasionally accompanied, music to those near the end of their life who feel that music could support them in this part of their journey. At a convenient time for all, some or all of us will come to the person's home to offer a session of music, during which families and loved ones are also welcome. We offer a range of music to match the support that is needed, including favourite song requests when possible."

It was her closing line that struck me: "I have wanted to do this kind of group singing work for the dying for a long time; it almost feels a bit like a calling."

Jessica is a music therapist by profession who specializes in caring for those with dementia and other chronic illnesses of aging. It's not as though she lacks opportunity to share music with people who are vulnerable and whose health is in decline. Yet here she was, feeling called to donate some of her talents and training to the dying and their families, over and above anything she might do to earn a living. Something special was happening here, and I wanted to find out more about a field that can elicit such commitment.

ONLINE GLIMPSES

Vignettes of Music Therapy in Action

"Hi, I'm Keegan. Or you can call me KJ for short," says the young man in black-framed glasses and a red golf shirt in the YouTube video. He calmly adds, "I have cerebral palsy and psychosis." Only his slightly laboured speech gives any hint of cerebral palsy. To my ear, he speaks gently and clearly. "I struggle to correct the false realities of my illness. I had puzzling thoughts, and when I concentrated too much those thoughts turned into nightmares."

I had almost passed over this video clip entitled "How Music Therapy Changed My Life," as I do many others that tout excessively the benefits of a particular therapy. (Prevent colon cancer by eating a dill pickle every day! Cure your back and shoulder pain with these three simple stretches!) However, the title lacked breathless punctuation and, more importantly, the source seemed legitimate. Children's Hospital Colorado, an academic pediatric hospital, evidently thought the video sufficiently important to have produced it professionally. The clip might have been short and simple, but the hospital had spent the money to do it well.

The scene switches to KJ sitting beside Tony, a music therapist, at a keyboard.

"Okay, so what's our thing?" Tony asks. "You had an idea."

"I think something jazzy."

"Jazzy. Do you mean happy jazz?" Tony plays a few bars.

"Yeah, happy jazz sounds good."

Tony transitions into an intro and then KJ, without cueing, launches softly into the song. "Stargazing in the moonlight. People dancing in the strobe lights…" His singing is both comfortable and competent.

The camera backs away as the music continues. KJ does a voiceover. "With Tony's help, I started to heal. Music takes me on a journey where I feel safe. I'm free to be myself, not what anybody else wants me to be."

One of the first comments about the video reads: "When he started singing, I got teary eyed. This is beautiful. I want to be a music therapist."

A few lines later, Pat wrote, "This YouTube by KJ is absolutely beautiful and inspiring. It gives hope to so many other children faced with so many challenges."

I can't say that I understood from the video how KJ's life had changed or how Tony had worked with him to reach that point, but, once again, I was intrigued. The scenario looked casual and ordinary, but perhaps it was this very normality that indicated an extraordinarily successful outcome.

I wanted to search for other YouTube videos that would give me a glimpse of therapists at work. The following presents some of what I found.

* * *

Ryan, perhaps in his thirties and wearing jeans and sneakers, casually cradles an acoustic guitar on his lap. Elliott is also seated, indifferently dressed in brown shorts and a tee-shirt. His age is hard to guess, but let's go with mid to late teens. Are they two brothers, two cousins, or just two friends hanging out?

What's peculiar is that they're in a sterile room, planted on folding metal chairs, face-to-face with their knees almost touching. As the video starts, Elliott rocks forward and then returns to an upright position. Forward and back, a cycle completed with each passing second. Elliott, it turns out, is autistic, and Ryan is his therapist.

"Hey, Elliott."

"Hello."

"How are you doing?"

"Good. How are you?"

"Good. So today we're going to start…"

"…with our Hello song."

"Yes. We're going to practise saying each other's name."

A caption appears on the screen, explaining that the purpose of the song is to rehearse using a person's name when greeting them.

Ryan explains, "I'll sing, 'Hello, Elliott.'"

"Hello, Elliott," Elliott echoes. This response might not be exactly what Ryan had in mind, but he lets it pass.

"And you will sing…"

"Hello, Elliott. Hello, Ryan."

"Yeah, 'Hello, Ryan.'" He doesn't point out Elliott's error, choosing instead to reinforce the correct portion of the response.

The strategy works. "Hello, Ryan," Elliott repeats. He's grasped the concept and the song can begin.

But not quite yet. Another caption appears, "We work on requesting by using motivating instruments."

Ryan continues, "And, Elliott, I've got all these instruments." He gestures grandly to half a dozen percussion instruments on the floor.

"Can I have the tambourine, please?"

"Nice asking, excellent." He reaches down and passes a plastic tambourine to Elliott. "Here you go."

Elliott shakes it a few times before saying thanks.

Ryan brings both hands to his guitar. "Alright, on a count of six."

As the song begins, another caption appears: "I match the rhythm of his rocking with my music in order to connect with him and honour his natural rhythm." Actually, Ryan does more than match the rhythm. He joins in the rocking, a very natural movement for a musical performer and sometimes even for the audience.

I hadn't given much attention to the swaying, but some of the commentators felt differently. "I adore that you actually went along with his stims! That would make me feel so much better in therapy if they acknowledged my stims, rather than pretending I'm not doing it."

"Exactly," added a viewer named Shepard, "because then they are acknowledging our emotions, essentially. Because that's what stimming is, processing emotions."

Barbara agreed. "Mirror technique helps to build bond and connection."

A little farther down the list of comments, Christine wrote, "Did you notice how the client stopped moving around as much towards the end of this video? Omg!"

The next song is accompanied only by both men clapping their hands together and on their laps, patty-cake style. "I control my body. I am in control. I'm calm, cool, collected, deep in my soul." Ryan occasionally interrupts the song, pausing to give Elliott a chance to practise controlling his body by also freezing for a second or two. Finally, he pulls back on his singing, the caption explains, to give Elliott the opportunity to sing the words independently.

Elliott's voice is less than melodious but Ryan encourages him, "Yeah, man, sing it." As the song ends, Ryan reaches out with each hand and shares a two-handed shake. Elliott seems fully engaged.

Next comes a requesting song, one that focuses on making choices, asking for things with full sentences, and using vocal inflection. A song they wrote together "to celebrate the strengths that Elliott has and to build his self-esteem" follows it. Not long afterwards, the caption draws my attention to a brief interaction that began with Ryan making a statement. His intent is to prompt a higher level of decision-making from Elliott than a question might.

The video ends with a whimper rather than a climax. I suppose that's the reality of most sessions. I did suspect, though, that not every session goes as well as the one I have just viewed.

Miss Molly had the same question. She wrote in the feedback section: "Has a client ever tried to grab the guitar from you or thrown an instrument? I ask because I play guitar and synthesizers and have been using some techniques like yours with my five-year-old son, who is autistic. He frequently wants to grab the guitar or bash the synthesizer keys—not angrily, he loves it, but gets too excited, I guess. I actually got him a cheap kid's guitar, and even gave him one of my old synths, but he always wants to 'take over' whatever instrument I'm playing or hit them out of excitement."

"Hey, Molly," Ryan replied, "I have that happen on a weekly basis! Good call on getting the cheap guitar. If he wants to take over an instrument, cool. Just grab a different one yourself, or do some body percussion or singing to accompany him. Follow his lead. You can also use sturdy percussive instruments like shape drums or floor drums. I hope that helps."

* * *

"Suppose I walked in," Hope E. Young says, after finishing her introduction, "and you were in a hospital. You're there because of suicidality, and you've just woken up in a psychiatric intensive care unit. You've just tried to kill yourself, and you're not real happy that you survived."

She explains that most people, when they're severely depressed, experience emptiness, or what's sometimes described as a hollow or Tin Man sensation. They've lost the ability to feel. Or sometimes they're angry, so very angry that they can feel nothing but anger. Hope says she is very careful not to play a happy song to a depressed person.

"That's called the iso-principle. I start where the person is. If that's sad or depressed, I'll usually start with sounds in a minor key, sad and slow. If they're angry, I might start with something loud and banging. Throwing things against the wall works really well. Banging a drum."

A few of the reviews of the video do a better job of conveying what she encounters in an angry person than she herself could probably describe:

— I yigh yigh…Jesus! This b.s. could push someone off a damn cliff. I mean, seriously. This was supposed to help.

— Her singing made me laugh so much. Laughing at, not with.

— Oh my god. If I were trying to kill myself, and a woman with a guitar walked in, she would probably regret it.

— She'd quit her job if she had to deal with me on my worst day.

— Talk to you would make me angry and aggressive and be filled to the brim with rage. But country music is what I listen to.

— This makes me more depressed. If she was in Kazakhstan, we would sell her to old man who handle sheep.

The comments about depression are more varied and nuanced. For example,

— Usually people who are depressed are very bottled up. I used to be a Tin Man, and the only time I felt anything was when I listened to music.
— People with depression sometimes need to hear the blues to remember they aren't alone. Seeing their own thoughts and feelings mirrored in music is validating and comforting.
— The song she played actually helped my depression. I got up every morning, coming to this video, and I fought it because of her.
— I would love to try this. One of the hardest parts of therapy is figuring out exactly how I feel, and why. Mostly I just feel like crap or sad, and I couldn't tell ya why.
— The talking made me feel worse, thanks.
— That's what I found so rewarding about working with music therapists. They helped me write out my feelings instead of just listening to music that made me more sad.

Hope's next topic is spirituality. "A lot of folks, even when they're depressed, are trying to connect with the spiritual." They might not feel connected to themselves or to a god of any kind, but they're thinking about it. "So spirituals are often a point where, if a person is sad and doesn't want to talk, I might just start playing something not very invasive. Something that's in the style of their preferences." She'll watch to see if the client relates to the music, if it has any meaning for them.

"Letting the music connect to people, and not having to say much, is a very powerful thing. From this point on, it's the patient. I may not play another note for the rest of the session. I might just sit quietly and let them connect with me, as they talk about themselves and I listen.

"I may take the song and allow them to put their own words into it." Hope demonstrates, strumming and singing, "I'm just a…" She pauses, saying she would now ask the client for words. After singing them, she'd check, "Does that feel right?" She seeks lyrics that enable her to become their instrument, which diminishes the Tin Man feeling.

"Sometimes so much emotion comes out that I have to try to use the music to contain that emotion so that they don't feel overwhelmed or their wounds reopen. The music can help the emotions grow and build, and then I move to resolve and leave them in what therapists call a closed position at the end of the session. Or, if they're about to work through trauma recovery, I might leave them open for a different kind of therapist or doctor to come in after me and do the deeper work."

✳ ✳ ✳

The television newscaster keeps the introduction short, in line with the brevity of the story itself. It's about using music in the treatment of substance abuse and addictions. I'm interested because it might hint at what happens in a group setting.

The clip begins with a young man, Cory, saying, "The whole group starts with a song. We introduce ourselves by name and how we're feeling that day. I've been with a guitar in this program, and I just start wailing away, getting everything out. Learning about myself."

A couple of scenes later, we finally hear from the therapist, Sheila. "I create and implement what we call music interventions, that the group works on. And the interventions always have the end goals in mind." These include minimizing loneliness, increasing concentration, and building a sense of community. "In the lyrics of a tune, we point out different life concepts, like forgiveness, overcoming challenges, remorse, or guilt. That will generate a group discussion."

Cut back to Cory. "It kind of gives me that extra push to get my thoughts out and on paper. Then I can bring them back into the group and we can discuss them."

* * *

The video opens with a singalong for a group of seniors. It's hard to tell that any of them are impaired. A woman with a guitar is seated at the front, where she has a clear view of each participant.

I immediately like the woman, Kerry, because she refers to the best plain English definition of music therapy I've encountered thus far: the use of music to achieve non-musical goals. She says that a lot of research has shown music helps the brain rewire itself around parts that are damaged. "That's one of the reasons that music therapy works."

"For this Parkinson's group," she continues, "we're focusing on using music to strengthen breath support and voice strength, as well as fine and gross motor movements. So you'll see some stretching and tapping to the rhythms." The secondary goals include self-esteem and mood improvement.

Parkinson's is a degenerative neurological disease with no cure at present. It affects everyone differently but is characterized by slow movements, rigidity, and tremors. I think of it as gradually losing control of one's body, even though I know a few mental processes are also sometimes weakened. About one percent of the population over age sixty is afflicted—a small proportion, but over a million North Americans live with Parkinson's disease or related disorders, known collectively as parkinsonism.

The singing presented in this clip, a pleasant but not memorable tune, proceeds at a moderate tempo, with Kerry strumming along in unobtrusive accompaniment. This low-key approach makes sense in that she's not there as a performer. During a break, the group does a little stretching, along the lines of chair yoga.

"With Parkinson's disease, it's almost like people have lost some of their internal rhythm, so some parts of the body stop moving the way they used to. By listening to music with a steady beat, and practising these things, we're hoping to compensate for that loss." This explanation helps me understand why a few participants have percussion instruments.

Looking at the scene from a less medical point of view, the session is a social activity for people who share the experience of living with Parkinson's disease. "Usually they don't want to leave after the class has ended, because they want to visit with each other."

The video closes with the host from the health care centre saying that exercise and music therapy can be as effective as drugs in helping some patients with their motor skills. Few people have commented on this video, but Stan took the time to write: "I have PD and it is quite the experience. Speech is one of my special interests. I'm concerned with swallowing down the road. We sang in our last LOUD Crowd class." This class, I later learned, is part of a vocal program for the ninety percent of people with Parkinson's at risk of developing a weakened voice and speech and swallowing difficulties.

∗ ∗ ∗

The spotlight shines harshly on Karla, who is standing alone on the stage. She's describing her youth, starting at age seven. "There was no one to tell and no one to ask for help, knowing and believing that if I did, my family would fall apart. And what would be worse would be finding out that my mother hated me. So it was up to me to make him stop."

While Karla was lying in bed one evening, her mother's piano playing transformed her, for a brief moment, from despair into feeling alive. Eventually the music ended and Karla drifted off to sleep. The music may have stopped, but her stepfather's abuse didn't.

Karla recounts looking for that piece of music a year or two later, desperately hoping to rekindle its life-giving energy. She eventually found it, but nothing happened the first time few times she plunked it out. It took until age ten for her to figure out that if she played the piece the way she felt in the moment, music could become a safe place to express herself. "So suicide was no longer the only option for escape."

Finally, at age nineteen, Karla disclosed the cause of her anguish and her family did indeed disintegrate. But she survived and is now a music therapist who understands how trauma can block one's ability to think and act. Music can provide an alternate route for building strength and developing the control to move forward.

A comment on one of the websites where the video appears concerns the healing power of music, even when only listening passively rather than actively producing it. "This talk has brought me so much understanding about my drive and need for certain songs to be played over and over again when my anxiety is most unbearable. Until now, I had no insight to why I obsessively listen to the same songs, only that it helps soothe me."

* * *

In another video, Kelly describes clients who have been triggered into trauma. "They can't calm down; they can't take a breath," she says. Their behaviour can seem histrionic to laypeople, given that the original event or causes may be long past, but it is not surprising to those knowledgeable about trauma.

Kelly uses a variety of techniques with people suffering such intense pain, with one particular method often proving effective. "I'll take the singing bowl and I just play that one tone for five, ten, fifteen minutes. I'll talk to them, sing a simple melody to them overtop the singing bowl. I'll say, 'Just keep trying to inhale.'"

I thought about my own fascination with wetting my finger and running it around the rim of a goblet to explore the types of sound I can generate. Kelly explains that the vibration of the bowl is like a musical massage: "If I'm working with somebody who was abused, touching them will make them feel worse. Human touch is too traumatic, too scary, and not trustworthy, but the vibrations of the singing bowl are completely safe." It's the vibrations that touch the person, helping them calm down sufficiently to begin breathing slowly and deeply, which in turn stimulates the vagus nerve to tell their body it's okay to de-stress.

"Then maybe they can start singing with me. It's just really simple singing, not even a song, most of time." She demonstrates with a long *ahh*, then repeats it at a lower pitch. "Once they're finally starting to get back in their body, and in the present, then we can start talking and problem solve and figure out what they need to express about their frightening place. How to be grounded so that they feel safe enough to walk out the door."

NEUROSCIENCE

I came to this chapter's topic unintentionally. Of all the videos promoting the benefits of music therapy, it was Erin's title, *Why I Want to Change the World with Music Therapy*, that happened to catch my attention one evening.

She starts broadly, commenting on the role of emotions and psychological well-being in physical health. Unsurprisingly, she claims music therapy fosters a more encompassing approach to health care and reminds us that its purpose is to bring about change. "The primary goals in the therapy are never musical," she says. "They might be the same goals as those in another therapy."

Then she shifts to a discussion of the brain and the means by which it processes music. The more scientists learn about these mechanisms, the more effectively therapists can harness them as a tool for transformation. So rather than the big-picture discussion of holistic health that I expected, Erin invites us to consider some specifics of brain physiology. I accept her invitation.

She emphasizes that music can be therapeutic because it is such a complex phenomenon, activating multiple parts of the brain. "When you boil everything down," she says, "music is one of the only things in life that processes information on both sides of the brain at once." Rather than a single musical lobe, the numerous components of music—such as melody, rhythm, pitch, and sometimes words—are processed in different parts of the brain.

"Because music uses both sides of the brain at once, when an area of the brain is damaged, or decreased—like with Alzheimer's disease, another area of the brain will try to make up for that loss. Through the use of music, the brain might be able to access a memory using a different neural pathway."

Oh, alternative pathways in the brain. Now that is *important. Really important.*

By way of example, the next videos I viewed showed an almost miraculous change in patients with dementia as they listen to the familiar music of their past. They not only brighten and sing, but some begin to engage with family members they barely acknowledged a few minutes earlier. I don't know if these individuals are typical of the dementia clients that therapists routinely encounter, but the clips nevertheless provided impressive instances of music activating different pathways in the brain. I later saw clients with Parkinson's dancing gracefully and no longer lurching, to illustrate how music can be used to alter body movements.

Erin had started her rhythm example by talking about the way a musical beat will pull the brain into matching the pattern, a process known as entrainment. Biologists define entrainment as the synchronization of organisms to an external perceived rhythm. The word "perceived" is important because sometimes the rhythm is inferred, meaning that the brain inserts it into gaps in the actual sound pattern. This ability to create rhythm, and not merely respond to it, is the key to some music therapy techniques.

Take, for example, a person who has had a stroke and whose walking has been affected. Walking is a rhythmic activity, but their brain has lost its ability to generate an internal rhythm to guide leg motion. Music becomes an external source of rhythm to pilot their feet. Eventually, if all goes well, the repetitive practice of pacing to music builds new pathways and perceived rhythm within the brain, which help the patient learn to walk independently.

I hadn't intended to look into the physiological underpinnings of music therapy because a few presentations I had seen in the past about the wonders of the brain dwelt excessively on anatomical details and provided too few applications of brain plasticity. Erin caused me to revise my thinking, and this chapter is the result.

* * *

Next, I watched a couple of Australian videos about music and the brain, one of which was a half-hour documentary by the Australian Broadcasting Corporation. I've elaborated some comments in it with a few excerpts from a TEDx talk in Perth. These two videos, along with the others I've drawn upon to write this book, are listed at the end. I'd encourage you to view a few of them for a fuller picture than the highlights I'm presenting.

The documentary began with a question that is at the heart of music therapy: Why is music so emotional, so memorable, and so powerful that it can revitalize a person even when much of the brain is damaged? The explanation, insofar as we have one, emerged from a series of interviews with individual scientists. To condense the information, I'm going to pretend that three such scientists came together in a panel.

"Let's start with what we know from neuroscience about the relationship between music and the emotions," June, the moderator of the imaginary panel, might have begun.

"Well," Alan responds, "music activates regions in the brain that are also activated when you perform co-operative, altruistic acts." These are acts where you look out for others or put their welfare ahead of your own.

June wrinkles her brow. "Okay, but I'm not seeing why this is inherently emotional."

Alan looks perplexed, as if the relationship should be obvious. Maggie jumps in: "Let's step back and come at this from a different angle. Music taps into deeply hardwired responses to certain vocalizations. Across the animal kingdom, alert calls tend to be high pitched, loud, and fast. Calming signals are lower pitched, soft, and slow. In humans, these basic tropes have become an entire, sophisticated language of emotion." June's face brightens as she slowly nods.

Another panellist, Marcel, picks up on the animal example. He explains that when primates bond through grooming, endorphins and oxytocin—feel-good hormones—are released to cement social bonds chemically. As only a limited number of monkeys can be groomed in a day, humans evolved to use music to release these hormones on a wider scale. Music became a vehicle for sharing emotion and forming social bonds.

Alan sees how to explain his original comment: "Oxytocin is well known to be associated with empathy, trust, and relationship building. The level of oxytocin in the bloodstream is raised when people are singing together, particularly when they are improvising." He adds that group music-making reduces sensitivity to pain as well as levels of the stress hormone cortisol.

June summarizes the role of music in the evolution of humans as a function without which we may never have become fully human. "It's all about bonding and the co-operative acts essential for societies to function." She asks if anybody can provide additional insights from evolutionary biology.

Marcel leans forward. "Many people believe," he says in a deliberate manner, "myself included, that music evolved from an earlier system that was largely just an emotional form of communication, an emotional proto-language." By way of evidence he cites the way that adults talk to babies, where pitch is exaggerated in simple speech. The overlapping areas of the brain for processing language and music suggest that perhaps the two evolved from a common precursor.

The conversation continues, veering off into the anatomical differences associated with music and language. It's Maggie who returns to the original question of why music is so emotional. "So, back in prehistory at some point, this proto-language split into language, which carried more information, and music, which continued to carry the message of emotion." She concludes that music is in some ways primal, predating even language.

Let's abandon my imaginary panel and return to two actual sequences in the ABC documentary, one about the mind and one about the body. The documentary asked how it is that music can penetrate the thick fog of dementia, doing something that no other stimulus is able to do. How does music serve as a side door into the brain, enabling patients with dementia—who are typically withdrawn—to come alive for a moment and reconnect with family members?

It turns out that we've already heard part of the answer, namely that music triggers both memories and emotions simultaneously. "It's like a super stimulus," an interviewee says. "So much of your brain is involved, there's more opportunity for the effects of music to be preserved in the face of damage." He adds that another consideration is sheer repetition. "Not only do we hear music verbatim, over and over, in a way that is unique and doesn't happen with speech, but we also imagine music—we hear it in our heads. It becomes deeply engrained, or tattooed, into the mind."

The narrator closes the Alzheimer's sequence by noting that music can sometimes calm the agitation of confused, stressed individuals who shout or act out, providing an alternative to psychoactive drugs.

As well as stimulating our mental processes, music is hardwired to make us move. Even as toddlers, we respond to music with our bodies. The ability to pick up a beat and move to it provides a clue as to why music can be used to unfreeze people and get them moving again.

In the video, the scene switches to a small dance studio where a therapist is helping a woman with Parkinson's jerk and shuffle her way to the centre of the floor. Then the music starts, and the therapist slides from the patient's side to face her. The pair assume a classic ballroom dance position. Soon they are gliding fluidly around the room.

"So what we think music does," the narrator wraps up, "is to bypass defective basal ganglia to activate what is trapped inside. The music provides an external rhythm to compensate for the defective rhythm inside the brain."

* * *

The morning drizzle had ended, but the clouds continued to hang low and close. Joggers and dog walkers dominated the shoreline path, with only the first of the baby strollers and children on scooters evident. As we sauntered along, Brendan asked if I was writing anything at the moment.

"Sort of," I replied. "I'm toying with the idea of doing something about music therapists. It's a field that's not very well known, and yet full of human interest. I know it's a good topic, but I'm still trying to figure out whether I'm capable of pulling it off. Mostly I've been exploring online, with the hope of eventually doing some interviews." His face brightened as he mentioned that he, too, was interested in how music affects the brain. We chatted along these lines for a few minutes, then moved on to other matters.

A text message chirped the next morning while I lay in bed, well before breakfast. Brendan had written: "Hi, Bob. Such interesting discussion on your interest/research in music and the brain. These are a few books in my collection on the subject. If you get the opportunity to read them, they are quite interesting."

From his collection? I thought. *Maybe he should be the person writing this book, not me.*

Brendan had photographed the covers of three paperbacks, one of which was Oliver Sacks' *Musicophilia: Tales of Music and the Brain*. "Tales" was an apt word, for the book consisted largely of case studies of musical oddities: musical savants, people who experience musical hallucinations, rhythm deafness, absolute pitch, associate colours or tastes with musical keys, and so on. Skimming through the book, I didn't learn as much as I desired about how the brain processes music but was struck nonetheless by this professor of neurology and psychiatry's high regard for music. "There is little doubt," he wrote, "that regular exposure to music, and especially active participation in music, may stimulate development of many different areas of the brain. Music can be every bit as important educationally as reading and writing."

Although we live in a musically saturated society—some people might hear more tunes in a month than their ancestors heard in a lifetime—I wonder whether active participation in music is actually declining. An emphasis on listening to professional performances, especially given the ease of downloading entire music libraries, seems to be displacing homegrown musical entertainment. Sacks did calm my related disquiet, though, that too many people may have missed the opportunity to learn how to make their own music. Unlike the early years of life when our brains are sponges for learning language, success in developing musical capacity is less age-dependent.

He pointed out that the neuroscience of music is only a little over half a century old, having emerged publicly in 1977 with Macdonald Critchley and R.A. Henson's book, *Music and the Brain*. Then, with the advances in brain imaging in the 1990s, medicine began to learn all sorts of things pertinent to music therapy, including the discovery of small anatomical differences in the brains of professional musicians compared to the rest of us.

One of the threads in Sacks' numerous tales concerned speech. The right hemisphere of the brain, which generally does only basic language processing, can be rewired in less than six months to become fairly capable linguistically. Music is the catalyst for this adaptation, starting with the therapist and patient singing a simple sentence. Then the musical elements of melody and rhythm are gradually removed, until only speech is left. A variation of singing is sometimes used to treat stuttering, because almost all people who stutter can sing fluently and freely. Here the trick is to help the stutterer envisage their speech as following a musical pattern.

In speech rehabilitation, a comfortable rapport between the client and music therapist may be crucial. This is because when we first learn to talk, the process is social as well as cognitive: a connection between our parents and us. Sacks contrasted the interpersonal chemistry needed in language recovery with a more aloof style of music therapy for certain types of movement disorders, where the music itself activates the motor system. "But with speech disorders like aphasia, the therapist and her relationship with the patient—a relationship which involves not only musical and vocal interaction but physical contact, gesture, imitation of movement, and prosody—is an essential part of the therapy. This intimate working together, this working in tandem, depends on mirror neurons throughout the brain."

A second thread to interest me the first time Sacks mentioned it was about movement, an attraction arising from my pleasure in already knowing the meaning of entrainment—the human tendency to keep time, to make motor responses to rhythm. My chest puffed out a little. I might have known a smidgen about entrainment, but it turned out to be less than I thought. Research has now shown that what seem to be our responses to rhythm actually precede the external beat. He noted, "We anticipate the beat, we get rhythmic patterns as soon as we hear them, and we establish internal models or templates. These internal templates are astonishingly precise and stable." Because entrainment involves the imagination and is not simply a response to a stimulus, I inferred that this is why rhythm is such a powerful tool in music therapy.

Sacks didn't dissuade me. I learned that thinking about music or rhythm may be as powerful, neurally, as actually listening to it. He described how rhythm, especially in smooth music, helps stimulate and synchronize movement. In contrast, he said, "Staccato, percussive music might have a bizarre counter effect, causing the patient to jump and jerk helplessly with the beat, like a mechanical doll or marionette."

He noted that while the tick of a metronome can help patients with their mobility, their walking would likely lack the fluency of a normal gait. To walk naturally, a continuous stream of stimulation is needed, with clear rhythmic organization. He added that dance is an ideal combination of music and movement, quite apart from its social benefits.

A third thread that interested me in *Musicophilia* involved dementia. Music therapy helps with this condition because musical perception and memory outlast other types of memory. The goal of music therapy with clients who have dementia is broader than for motor or speech disorders, namely to help people reclaim their identity. "It aims to enrich and enlarge existence, to give freedom, stability, organization, and focus."

To illustrate what he meant by a broader purpose, Sacks reproduced a letter from an Australian music therapist, Gretta, who worked with people with dementia living in a nursing home. She wrote that, at first, she thought she was just providing entertainment but came to see herself as a can opener for memories. "One of the loveliest outcomes of my work is that nursing staff can suddenly see their charges in a whole new light, as people who have a past, and not only a past but a past with joy and delight in it." As for the clients, "There are always people who cry. There are people who dance, and people who join in." In addition to bringing a flicker of sunshine into sometimes dreary settings, Gretta simultaneously tackles a few deeper concerns. "There are disturbed people who become calm, and silent people who give voice, frozen people who beat time. There are people who don't know where they are but who recognize me immediately as 'the Singing Lady.'"

The videos I had seen about nursing homes usually involved residents listening to music or singing with the therapist. Sacks mentioned drum circles, an additional technique for people with dementia. These circles can be valuable because, like dance, drumming activates primitive parts of the brain.

With chronic movement disorders, as distinct from the rehabilitation of injuries, patients usually revert to their usual movement patterns as soon as the music stops. The emotional benefits and physical strengthening might endure, but the movement gained while listening to music evaporates instantly. In contrast, the improvements in patients with dementia can last for hours or days. Eventually, though, the patients return to their original physical state. It's their friends and relatives who benefit long term from seeing their loved ones respond to music.

Much of what Sacks described was not the intentional use of music to achieve a non-musical goal. In other words, he wrote relatively little about music therapy. His outpouring of stories affirmed the many and varied ways that music affects all of us, to lesser or greater extents, in particular situations. He happened to emphasize the greater extents, the seemingly incredible stories. Music may even, at times, "resist the distortions of psychosis and be able to penetrate the deepest states of melancholia or madness, sometimes when nothing else can."

* * *

I obtained the two Daniel Levitin books that Brendan recommended from my local library. They taught me a lot about music and its role in society but little about its therapeutic use. A statement near the beginning of *This Is Your Brain on Music* brought to mind the lines I'd seen about the lack of ego in music therapy. "Only relatively recently in our culture, five hundred years or so ago," he wrote, "did a distinction arise that cut society in two, forming separate classes of music performers and music listeners. Throughout most of the world and for most of human history, music-making was as natural an activity as breathing and walking, and everyone participated." Maybe therapists should be in the vanguard of helping all of us recover something we're losing, namely the ability to make music ourselves for the sheer joy of it, as neither a performer nor a listener.

One sentence Levitin wrote about an African language encapsulated why music therapists so often join health teams that treat movement disorders and injuries: "The Sesotho verb for singing, *ho bina*, as in many or the world's languages, also means to dance. There is no distinction, since it is assumed that singing involves bodily movement." In our Western culture, we do make this distinction, and perhaps, as with the performer-listener distinction, we are the poorer for it.

Along with treating ailments of the body, music therapists also tend to patients with emotional challenges. Unfortunately, as of 2008 when Levitin wrote *The World in Six Songs*, "understanding why it is music and not something else that causes these strong feelings of social bonding remains partly a mystery."

This news deflated me, but then I recalled how young the field of brain and mind research really is. Not only is it new, few of its researchers focus on the brain's processing of music. "The field of music cognition is relatively small," Levitin wrote. "There are probably only two hundred and fifty people in the world who would consider it their speciality. Contrast this with a field like neuroscience, which draws 30,000 attendees to its annual conferences in the United States alone." Give us time and give us people, Levitin seemed to be saying, and we'll unlock more secrets of the brain, keys to helping us use music to restore and maintain the health of the people we love.

BECOMING A THERAPIST

The Asian American woman in the video doesn't give her name, but some of the viewer comments are addressed to RubatoMT, who posted the clip. It's probably a pseudonym because *rubato* is a musical term that instructs the performer to be expressive and flexible with the rhythm. The literal translation from the Italian is "stolen," as in stealing a smidgen from a beat or bar to give to another one.

Rubato appears to be in her late twenties, with shoulder-length hair and a disarming smile that she flashes regularly. During her teenage years, she says she dreamed of joining a professional orchestra and travelling the world. Her instrument? The clarinet. She was good enough to gain admission to a music conservatory after finishing high school.

"The second I got there," she confesses, "I realized it wasn't going to be what I thought. I felt pretty lost." She's not the first college student to have had that disappointment, but, unlike many, she persisted with her studies.

During a visit with her family in second year, her mother asked whether music therapy might be an alternative to performing in an orchestra. Rubato had never considered this career for herself, although she knew of acquaintances from high school who were pursuing it. A seed had been planted.

As fate would have it, her conservatory offered an introductory music therapy course that she could use as an elective in her program. "I took it, kind of on a whim. That was probably the first time that I realized there is more to music than just the final product. Music therapy reminded me why I loved music in the first place." She explains that while working so hard to become a proficient performer, one who learns quickly and can consistently deliver a good product, she had lost the enjoyment of simply making music, regardless of how polished the session might be. The music therapy course helped her recover her appreciation of the creative process, as well as the friendships that can develop along the way.

This observation resonated with me. I recalled one of my daughter's piano teachers inexplicably encouraging her to enter a music festival. Rarely, outside a funeral or protest demonstration, have I witnessed a less festive venue. What was termed a festival was, in truth, an examination or competition where nervous children were judged and found mostly not to have achieved the gold standard. Pedagogies have since changed, but in earlier times I suspect formal music lessons put as many kids off music as turned them on to it.

In the video, I noticed Rubato shifting her comments away from herself and towards others. "I truly believe that everyone is musical," she says. "It's not whether you're good. It's about being creative and having fun together. Everybody has a connection to music, even when we don't have the words to describe how we're feeling." She adds, "Music therapy has taught me a lot about courage."

How so? I wondered.

"Every day, I ask my clients to do something they may never have done before. I think my biggest problem with performing had been my own fear, my own vulnerability. Every day, my clients show me that there's nothing to be scared about."

* * *

What sorts of people become music therapists? I pondered. *And how might I find out?* It finally dawned on me that a data set I had encountered in my work life might give me a few clues.

All public colleges and universities in British Columbia survey their former students about their educational experiences, as well as to find out what the grads did in the year or two after finishing their program. The surveying has its quirks, but, on the whole, it's a good source of information. Even though not all music therapists in British Columbia studied at Capilano University, Capilano's survey results could begin to answer my question.

The music therapy report I tracked down included just over fifty respondents, an acceptable number from a statistical point of view. The response rate was also decent, with fifty-seven percent of those eligible for the survey having completed it. There was still a chance that certain types of graduates had declined to participate—those embarrassed about being unemployed, for example—and had thereby biased the results, but any bias would be small because of the high response rate. Governments and businesses often have to make do with far less robust data than these.

I wasn't at all surprised that eighty-five percent of the respondents were female. Society may be less sexist than a generation ago, but men are still overrepresented in occupations that involve working with things, while women staff so many of the caring professions that serve people.

The music therapy students were a little older than the typical Capilano student. Based on their age at the time of the survey, it appeared that a fair number had been in their late twenties or early thirties when they entered the music therapy program (in their third year at university). Just as many must have continued their studies quite soon after leaving high school, perhaps taking a part-time course load for the first couple of years. A sprinkling of older students rounded out the sample.

The graduates were happy with the curriculum and how Capilano delivered it to them. Their satisfaction level was a little above the university average, but more telling was the statistic that ninety-two percent would select the same program again. As is common, one-quarter continued studying after graduation, mainly in master's programs or to obtain some sort of professional certification.

On the employment front, virtually all the respondents had entered the labour force successfully, with their unemployment rate sitting at less than five percent. The vast majority were working in their field. What caught my attention was that a slight majority were self-employed, often working multiple part-time jobs. Earnings were in line with those of recent grads from other Capilano bachelor's programs, but the potential for income growth wasn't clear—salaries in some fields start low but increase significantly over time, whereas those in other fields plateau quickly.

I found this statistical snapshot helpful, but it didn't tell me anything about the respondents' motivations for becoming—and remaining—music therapists. To learn about that topic, I would have to talk to people, and so I began making inquiries.

* * *

I returned to Rubato, my new YouTube friend. I wanted to learn about her internship, the last step in the training to enter the profession. She rewarded my faithfulness in the next video by revealing her real name. It's Mai. I also learned that her practice in San Jose is at Creative Vibes.

In the video, Mai sits in the same room as the earlier video, although it seems a touch more organized than I remembered. A glass-paneled door, each panel framed in natural wood, features to her right. To her left, various musical props rest on a built-in shelf, hovering well above the corner of a laminate table and below a wall-mounted speaker. The ambience is professional and warm.

Part of Mai's presentation consisted of advice about financial planning for the half-year internship—a typical concern of students, but not my interest. I was drawn, instead, to her comments about therapy sessions in real life differing from practice ones.

"One of the things I struggled with during my internship," Mai recalls, "was learning how to be spontaneous and flexible, while still creating a safe and productive environment for my clients. In school, I wrote out exactly what I was going to say, and exactly how the session would go. But people and life are totally unpredictable. I discovered that sometimes my clients had very different needs than I had initially thought. This sent me into a panic, and I didn't know what to do."

Mai gradually realized that her desire to plan for every contingency arose from a fear of doing poorly in a session. She learned that planning was not nearly as important as having the skills to adapt. "The day I took a leap and started being okay with flexibility was the day that I began connecting in a genuine and authentic way with my clients. Even when things…"—here she makes air quotes with her fingers, as she says the words 'fall apart'—"that's an opportunity for you to explore."

Ruefully she elaborates, "There are no step-by-step directions for how to handle situations like when a client tries to grope you, or when a client threatens physical violence to another client in the middle of a group. It's okay not to have all the answers."

She pauses and stares intently at the camera. "It's okay," she says, nodding in emphasis. Another pause, and she slowly finishes, "What matters is that you're authentic and honest, because this will help your clients to be the same with you, and with others."

* * *

Having already scanned the structure of one university's music therapy program, I wondered whether all schools take similar approaches in preparing students to enter the profession. Simply because it had been in the news recently a midwestern city came to mind as a potential place to make a comparison. Not a bad idea, I decided, as it is the home of a well-respected university. So I took a peek online, and the university does indeed offer a music therapy program. It's a self-contained four-year program that contrasts with the two-years-plus-two-years model at Capilano University.

I could be off base, but that midwestern university's curriculum seems to reflect the view that a good grounding in classical music makes it possible, when the need arises, for a graduate to slide readily into other genres, such as jazz, country, or pop. It also appears that the program's graduates emerge much stronger in music than in psychology and physiology. Not all music therapy programs share this emphasis, but that's okay—some variation among schools widens the path towards new understandings and techniques.

My first impression—shaped, no doubt, by my background as an education bureaucrat—was that this midwestern university's music therapy program is the offspring of an established music program and was developed on the existing strengths of the faculty, rather than being designed from scratch. Drawing heavily upon current courses and expertise is, after all, usually the cheapest and easiest way for a postsecondary institution to launch a new program.

Take, for example, the requirement of three courses about the history of western music, a common requirement in classical music programs. The first of these courses includes the Medieval and Renaissance periods—helpful, I suppose, for therapists working with clients who like listening to Gregorian chant. Adding therapy students to an existing history class for performance students, if indeed the university does this, boosts revenue from tuition fees and from any enrolment-based grants provided by the government. The best part is that the costs of accommodating the extra students can be minimal, perhaps little more than hiring an assistant once in a while to help with the additional marking. Combining students from multiple programs in a shared course, in order to create economies of scale, is a tried-and-true strategy for strengthening a school's finances.

Now, my over-active imagination took off, focusing on the practical, and even cynical, aspects of academic life. I envisaged a curriculum design committee, deep in conversation, planning a new music therapy program for some fictitious university.

"Therapists sometimes have to lead groups of clients," one member of my imaginary committee observes. "You know, having them sing or drum. It's not all about playing for clients, or one-on-one work."

"Yeah, you're right. So what do we do? Our budget is tight."

"Why not throw them into our conducting course? Leading a drop-in group of patients with Parkinson's in some songs can't be all that different from directing a mixed choir or a chamber ensemble. It would keep timetabling simpler than adding a new course just for therapy students."

"That makes more sense than putting them into a course for keyboard accompanists."

Next, I pictured the worst of the personnel considerations that might form the backdrop for this imaginary curriculum committee.

"If we end up with a few therapy instructors who are more comfortable in a blues bar than the opera house, we'll still have to invite them to the Christmas party and give them a vote at departmental meetings. There's a risk to hiring people who specialize in non-orchestral instruments, such as the accordion or banjo. They might not have the same values and priorities as us. Much safer to stick with people who resemble us, and can prepare our grads to enter clinical settings with an oboe or French horn in hand."

"I agree. In a similar vein, let's up our audition requirements for program admission to at least eight years of piano and three years of lessons in voice or another instrument. That should help screen out any riffraff who have honed their musical skills in a garage band."

* * *

"No kidding," I blurted. "You teach music therapy—and not in the jazz program?" A new energy infused my casual exchange with this stranger as we awaited the passenger ferry that crosses Vancouver's harbour. Rosilyn, I had just learned, was a faculty member at Capilano University.

I described my music therapy project. "I write this type of creative non-fiction because I love hearing the in-depth stories of real people." She remained receptive but noncommittal when I suggested my book might eventually be a good orientation for prospective students, and even promotional material for potential employers. *Fair enough,* I thought, *she has no idea whether I write well or how I'm approaching the subject.*

I asked what her students find the more challenging aspects of their training and said I gathered that learning how to improvise can be a big leap for some musicians. She grinned.

She said that despite sharing core values, the instructors have very different styles and approaches. The students have to learn to adapt, rather than use the same essay format or study techniques in all their classes. "I remind them that people are complex. Students need to experience a variety of approaches because clients are all different. When students resist this rationale, wanting to be told the one best way to do things, there's usually a reason in their history why they crave certainty.

"Some struggle with disclosing about themselves when they're not used to it, or they try to stay below the radar and not say a lot. I've learned that some painfully quiet people can be really good in the field when they're on practicum, so I try not to fixate on how much they participate in class. But I still need some evidence that they're engaged and making progress. Teaching and learning is tough with scant feedback."

She rubbed her hand over her chin. "It's a very stressful program, exciting and exhausting. Students are loving it, and crying, and dealing with their own histories all at once. Some who don't even stay in music therapy after graduating still swear by their training because it made them better human beings."

I asked if that intensity means there are strong bonds among those who remain in the profession, given that over half the local therapists have gone through the Capilano program.

"I would say so, especially because it's taught as a cohort. Students take almost all their classes together for two years." She added that she had expected less group closeness when the program had to shift online during the COVID-19 pandemic, but that really hadn't been the case. "It did kind of wreck making music together, though."

We continued chatting as the ferry—a blue-and-white catamaran—eased into its slip and discharged passengers through the automatic doors on the far side of the vessel. Next, the doors on our side opened, allowing us to step onboard. With fewer than a hundred people boarding, and only a handful more striding down the passageway, Rosilyn and I easily found adjacent seats. I placed my knapsack on the seat beside me, pleased not to have to rest it on my lap.

"My biases notwithstanding," Rosilyn said, "I do think Capilano's is one of the best programs in North America. It differs from those that have a performance or classical emphasis. Cap's students get lots of practical experience and develop great people skills. We have applicants who identify as being a singer-songwriter. They don't have Grade 10 piano or classical guitar, but they may have raw talent chops that will serve them really well. We'll accept them when many programs won't."

"But how do they fare after they leave you?" I asked. "Sometimes the world isn't ready for what one has to offer."

"Quite nicely, thank you very much. Our graduates get snatched up for internships and jobs across Canada. It's less so the other way around. We're more process oriented than many schools."

"Process oriented? What does that mean?"

"Things like counselling skills and understanding yourself as a practitioner. What makes you tick and issues you haven't worked through that might show up with clients. Like how can you be available for clients in a nursing home if you're still mad at your grandfather and one guy there reminds you of him?"

"But where does the product fit in? Surely a therapist has to be a decent musician and actually achieve something with the client."

"Oh, for sure. We'll fail students if they can't play well enough. It's just that I don't see the value in making students learn things like obscure musical terms, often in Italian, that they'll never use in a therapeutic setting."

Rosilyn peered at me, as if assessing whether she could say more. She eventually claimed her program's willingness to fail students is a strength. "I don't know if all other schools do that, once the student has met their entrance requirements. At our place, you could reach the last semester and still fail, especially practicum. There's quite a high bar."

Sometimes students are encouraged to drop back to a partial course load, to free up time so that they can work on their musical or other deficiencies. But sometimes they are obliged to leave the program entirely. I asked how often that happens.

"In each of the past few years," she replied, "at least two people have been required to leave the program, out of a class of about twenty-one. In fourth year, we're usually down to sixteen people, due to dropouts and expulsions. Some of the reason may involve musicianship, but it's also due to character and maturity, especially relational. We have some students who are fantastic musicians but can't do the relationship piece and work with clients. So they don't do well in the program."

Rosilyn looked out a window. A little to the east, a twin propeller seaplane banked into its final descent, its ungainly pontoons tipped towards us. Like construction cranes, these low-and-slow aircraft routinely defy the laws of physics.

"How did you end up at Capilano?" I asked. "Did you practise music therapy for a while, or did you go straight into graduate school to get your advanced qualifications?"

It turned out that Rosilyn had worked in long-term care for a number of years before enrolling in a master's program in the humanities. "A lot of my colleagues were doing a master's in music therapy, but I thought that was too narrow. My thesis was about music and spirituality in dementia care."

"And did you need a doctorate to get on at Cap?"

"I eventually earned a PhD, this time in education, that focused on the creative arts and trauma. That's what opened up the opportunity for me to teach at Capilano."

"So you didn't do more music studies, beyond your bachelor's degree?"

"No."

I asked about the university's expectations for her to conduct research, the publish-or-perish mantra in the back of my mind.

"Well, I'm currently working on elements of a massive study about music therapy and Alzheimer's. It's a collaborative project funded by the Alzheimer Society of Canada and administered by the Division of Neurology at the University of British Columbia. And, of course, there are smaller, practice-based grants. I'm applying for one right now to study clients with adverse childhood experiences."

"What are practice-based grants?"

"They're designed to help frontline workers do a little research, often to assess the impact of some new initiative they're trying. Health authorities offer some. Even universities will provide a few thousand dollars here and there so that an instructor can hire a student to be a research assistant. I think the cost-benefit ratio is generally quite good. The grants tend to be a lot of work for the researcher, but they're interesting and contribute to the credibility of the field.

"Having to do some research reminds me of the appeal of music therapy," she concluded as we prepared to disembark at Lonsdale Quay. "On the surface, it seems simple. But to do it well, and to know what approach to take in particular situations, is not."

SNIPPETS FROM LAYPEOPLE

Lucia, a social services worker, and I met while volunteering in a demonstration garden at an environmental centre. I had moved on to other activities but we made a point of staying in touch. We were now chatting in a park, catching up on the past several weeks.

I mentioned meeting a music therapist who had figured out how to keep working during COVID by seeing her clients outdoors—masked, one on one, and socially distanced, of course. Lucia pressed her head forward ever so slightly. "Tell me about that," she requested. "A couple of my agency's clients have benefited from music in the past, and I'd like to learn about options during the pandemic."

I was eager, perhaps overeager, to respond, but chose to hold back. "Only if you'll tell me about your experiences first," I replied. "You serve only adults, not kids, right?"

"In my program, yes. Some are able to live on their own and hold a job, just needing somebody to check on them for an hour or two each week. Others need plenty of support. They're all developmentally disabled, but to varying extents."

"How has music helped them?"

"Well, the guy who springs to mind is middle-aged and non-verbal. His foster mother for the past three or four years is just lovely. She was the one who noticed that when he heard a favourite song on the radio, he'd occasionally sing a word or two. This didn't happen often, so it took somebody who was around him a lot, and paying attention, to notice."

"Did this mean he had some capacity to speak but wasn't using it?"

"Yes. At least, that's what the foster parents suspected. So a manager found a little money to get him into some sort of music therapy at the conservatory. I don't know the details, just that when he started, his attention would lapse after fifteen minutes. That's not much time for a therapist to accomplish anything."

"But, obviously, something good happened or you wouldn't be telling me this story."

"You're so perceptive," Lucia gushed, rolling her eyes. "It took months of weekly sessions, but they boosted his attention span to forty-five minutes and got him to say a few phrases. Usually he speaks only in response to a prompt, but sometimes he initiates."

"This is probably going to sound ignorant or heartless," I said, "but I don't see why that's a big deal. It's nice and all that, but it seems like a lot of effort for a relatively small payoff. What am I missing?"

"Don't feel badly about asking," she reassured me. "If you don't know our clientele, it can be hard to assess what's major and what's minor. The thing you need to remember about this particular client, who I'll call Hector, is that he has likes and dislikes, just as everybody does. And he naturally gets frustrated when he's repeatedly exposed to things he doesn't care for. Unlike us, though, he doesn't have the language to say what's wrong. So he often just lashes out when he's unhappy.

"This man is about six feet tall. He doesn't mean to do any harm, but if you're a skinny, twenty-year-old aide, it can be scary to accompany him. We have safety protocols in place and all that, but these just reduce the risk, not eliminate it."

"Oh," I said, "I'm starting to get it. Even a tiny vocabulary could be a big thing."

"Yes. Here's what happened at a social event called Namaste that Hector attends one afternoon each month. It's a live band concert held in the sanctuary of a big church. The venue is great because it's a totally controlled environment. Only people with disabilities and their caregivers attend, and all the caregivers watch out for whoever is around them, not just their own charges. Everybody is used to this population, so the atmosphere is relaxed. Our clients love the upbeat music and the freedom to sit or wander or dance and be themselves, however odd that might be. Actually, I've quite enjoyed it the few times I've attended.

"Well, on one occasion, for whatever reason, Hector decided partway through that he had had enough. 'Overwhelmed,' he told his caregiver. That's a pretty sophisticated word, but that's the one he used. His aide got the message right away and gently ushered him out. No fuss, no muss."

"You're suggesting he could have ignited a brawl in the days before music therapy?"

Lucia wrinkled her nose. "Probably not that serious, but perhaps sufficient to generate an incident report." She stopped and peered at me. "Imagine what it's like now that he can voice a few of his likes and dislikes, even if just occasionally. Imagine how much better that makes life for him and for us." She smiled. "Certainly for us, and I'm pretty sure for him as well.

"So was that money for his music therapy well spent?" she continued. "I think it was, if you compare it to the huge amounts spent elsewhere in health care and the human services for outcomes that may or may not be as long lasting or life changing."

I scooped some pebbles, lazily letting them slip through my fingers, while Lucia shifted over to a wider spot on the log. The breeze had picked up a little, filling the sails of the dinghies near the opposite shore. Their progress remained sluggish, but at least they were no longer becalmed.

I returned my gaze to Lucia and said, "You used to work with autistic people in your previous job, didn't you?" This was a rhetorical question. My real question came next: "Did you encounter music therapy back then?"

Lucia thought for a moment. "No, not all." She must have seen my disappointment because she added, "But I can recall one situation where some help from a speech or music therapist could have been quite valuable."

"I'm listening."

"Tori was a severely autistic teenager who had only a handful of words, so she used the same words to mean different things. Plus, she sounded kind of robotic. The sounds were clear, but because she lacked inflection and didn't use full sentences, it could be hard to know if she was asking a question, giving an order, or just making a statement. Anyhow, to give her an outing, we'd sometimes take her to watch amateur hockey in the evening. She enjoyed the game, and the bleachers were sufficiently empty that the crowd didn't overstimulate her.

"All would be well until late in the game when her aide might have to get her back to the group home for the 10:00 p.m. shift change. Tori would freak out, hollering and grabbing the edge of her seat. She even resisted our last-ditch efforts to bribe her with barbeque potato chips—she really liked junk food, and keeping her away from it was an ongoing challenge. Needless to say, she was a big girl.

"I was with her at a game where she kept saying, 'Go home. Go home.' I emphatically said no, we were staying until the end of the game, and this would quiet her for a while. Then she'd repeat, 'Go home.' This ticked me off because I knew that if we were to leave then, and not after the game ended, she'd have a hissy fit.

"Finally it dawned on me that she was asking a question. Were we about to leave? She was happy at the game and wanted reassurance that she could watch it all. Then, after the game had ended and she again said, 'Go home,' I realized she had switched to making a statement. She was telling me she was ready to go, and we left without incident.

"My point is that I hadn't realized how much I rely on intonation to understand the meaning of a phrase, and Tori didn't know how to use intonation. A small thing, but one with big implications until we figured it out. Unfortunately, inflection is a pretty complicated skill to try and teach even someone with a strong vocabulary."

I agreed. "Yes, I can see why you'd like a therapist who could help. But you'd still have to deal with the scheduled shift change if the game hadn't ended yet."

"The union was great," she replied. "The staff all agreed that the shift would end whenever the game ended, regardless of whether that was before or after 10:00. So it was a happily-ever-after outcome, especially as our team won a decent number of games."

Lucia stared at her feet. I surmised she was strolling down memory lane, and I seemed to have been correct. She said, "Tori's roommate, Natasha, was even lower functioning. Her single mother couldn't begin to cope with looking after her at home, especially after splitting up with her boyfriend. What's so sweet, though, is that the ex-boyfriend remained very good to Natasha. He continued to visit her every few weeks in the group home, bringing his guitar with him. Conversation was impossible, and music was one of the few ways he could connect with her. He knew what songs she liked, and could read her moods. I'm not sure who benefited the most."

* * *

Nattering during our weekly badminton sessions, my companions were showing more interest in my current writing project than I expected. They might not have known much about music therapy, but they vaguely sensed the topic was thought provoking and important. And every once in a while, somebody contributed a tidbit to my rapidly expanding knowledge base.

"My two uncles," Barry told me as he zipped his racquet into its softcover case, "have major hearing loss. Runs in the family. One is macho, denying his problem and refusing to get hearing aids. The other overcompensates, doing everything he can to cope with his loss. I was taken aback when I learned he was seeing a music therapist, along with a raft of audiologists."

"Music therapist?" Sandeep echoed. "Seems kind of contradictory. If you can't hear very well, why on earth would you want to do something that involves hearing? I get why a blind person might want a music therapist, but a deaf person?"

Barry plunked himself on the bottom bench of the bleachers. "I wondered the same thing. Though he's not totally deaf, just hard of hearing. Turns out he's not so unusual in going to a music therapist."

"Seriously?"

"Yeah. Apparently it has something to do with sharpening what hearing he still has, and helping prevent his speech from worsening—starting to slur or talk with an unusual cadence, I guess." Barry then changed the subject, asking if the tournament next week would bump us from our usual court time. But he had sparked my interest in the hard of hearing.

A few days later, I searched for websites describing music therapy for the hearing impaired. Part of the therapist's task in these situations, I learned, is simply motivational because developing careful attention to residual sounds is a complex and tedious process. Music is usually more accessible than speech, and making the occasional use of melody is more fun and rewarding than relying exclusively on spoken drills and exercises.

Another task for the therapist concerns the awkward or unnatural speech of some people with hearing impairments. "These individuals commonly lack the internal feedback mechanisms necessary for monitoring and adjusting, for instance, pronunciation of words, vocal inflection, or speech rhythm," explained one website. "They tend to demonstrate fewer variations in pitch and intonation than normal-hearing speakers, which results in a monotone. They often prolong syllables and/or sentences and frequently pause inappropriately." The bottom line is that the speech of those with impaired hearing can become progressively harder to understand as the years pass, adding to their social isolation.

Music can help develop these prosodic features of speech. The breathing, rhythm, pitch, and articulation needed to sing a song all reinforce the structures required for intelligible speech. Music therapists thus strengthen these expressive, or spoken, skills in addition to the client's receptive, or listening, abilities.

About three weeks after Barry described his relatives' hearing loss, Ying Yue sidled over to me during a badminton game we were both sitting out. She's a full-time library technician who is chipping away at a degree in applied psychology, taking one or two courses per semester. "What Barry said a while ago about his hard of hearing uncle interested me. So when a prof mentioned music therapy in a module about addictions and substance abuse in one of my courses, I paid more attention than I normally would. Would you like to hear what she said, or do you already know enough about the topic?"

"Tell me, please. I hardly know anything."

"It sounded rather lame at first. Feel-good stuff, I thought, about group bonding and reducing isolation, and expressing emotions. I could imagine some of the attendees rolling their eyes. Would beddy-bye stories be told, they might wonder? Some *kumbaya* moments? Then, as the instructor talked, it started making sense to me."

"How so?"

"In addition to a lot of lying and manipulating and denying to others, addicts also tend to develop a bunch of defence mechanisms to justify their behaviour to themselves."

"You mean rationalizations, like 'I wouldn't have got wasted if I hadn't been pressured to attend the party?'"

"Yes. Or minimizing problems or thinking others envy their lifestyle or a bunch of other things. The key point is that these defences can become so powerful that the person with the addiction loses touch with what they're actually feeling. Can you imagine a counsellor trying to have productive conversations with clients who can spin a good story but who are vague or mistaken about their own emotions? How do you identify a client's inner conflicts and blockages when their emotional awareness seems at times to be that of a preschooler?" I placed my racquet on the bench beside me, aware that my habit of spinning it might annoy others. Before Ying could comment on my compulsive behaviour, I asked if music's value in addictions is as a means for people to recognize and acknowledge emotions.

"Yes," she replied. "Music seems innocent and fun, in no way a threat to the rigid, self-perpetuating addictive system." She paused and gave a lopsided smile. "That last bit sounded like it came from a psych major. Did you understand the jargon?"

"Not entirely, but you impressed me."

"Here's an example. A person in rehab gets some one-on-one counselling, but there's also a lot of group work."

"Like in Alcoholics Anonymous?" I interjected.

"I suppose. We haven't covered A.A. in class. Just that developing positive relations with peers is important in a lot of treatments, but this is hard because addicts tend not to trust others and may be fairly isolated. Denying their problem, denying their inability to relate to others, and denying their own emotions: these are deep-seated coping mechanisms that resist change. The mechanisms might be dysfunctional, but they're the only ones the addicts have. So the early stages of recovery require some non-threatening techniques to work around those defences."

"Music therapy as a subversive activity?" I quipped.

Ying agreed. "That's pretty much right. Choosing a set of songs or rewriting lyrics lets an individual express themselves safely. You can talk about the pain in a sad song without sounding like a wimp yourself. You can say how much it sucks when the singer's friends let them down, without having to admit that you regularly do this to others. Music becomes a place to practise identifying emotions and expressing them. They're steps towards self-awareness and taking responsibility for addiction and recovery."

I started to say something about non-threatening ways to engage isolated or ashamed people when a shuttlecock landed at my feet. "Does this mean you've finished your game," I shouted to the players, "and it's our turn?"

As Ying and I rose to enter the court, she added that self-expression often precedes self-awareness. Then we dropped our discussion of music therapy in favour of more pressing matters.

Conversations

ANNETTE

"I was a little shocked," I admitted, "when I first heard music therapists talking about playing with clients. Not playing instruments, though of course that happens a lot. Just playing, in the everyday sense of the word. It conjured up images of goofing off and wasting time." Annette straightened in her patio chair, her green eyes widening. "Then I felt sheepish," I continued, "as I realized I had missed whole levels of meaning."

"Yes," she said, "playing is serious business. Developmental psychologists figured out ages ago that children use play to learn about themselves, explore roles, and test boundaries. Practise the give and take of relationships. Maybe even overcome previous limitations. In the same way, when we're using improvisational models of music therapy, there's a lot more going on than the casual onlooker might realize."

Annette relaxed her shoulders as I nodded in comprehension, but her posture remained guarded. She elaborated on the human need to explore and express oneself in a safe space, as well as to receive support and feedback from others. "These other people include the music therapist, of course, or fellow music-makers in a small music therapy group. And, I should add, don't underestimate the importance of a client experiencing wholeness instead of disability or illness."

We were chatting in her side garden, comfortably shaded as the summer sun dropped behind the horse chestnut trees that line the street. The National Hockey League had figured out how to hold playoffs during the COVID pandemic, and the occasional groan or cheer drifted from the living room where some of her family had gathered to watch a game. I'm not a fan of spectator sports, and apparently Annette isn't either, at least not of hockey.

I picked up on Annette's use of the word "explore." "I've come to realize that play is sometimes used to mean exploring or experimenting with the client. Kind of like a schoolteacher trying to figure out what approaches will work best with kids who have different learning styles."

"Yes," she said carefully, as if she wasn't entirely convinced I was heading down the best path. "As music therapists, we need to observe and assess. Some techniques have standardized assessments, but first we develop a relationship with the client. We usually do that through music, and we gradually figure out which approaches might work best."

"When I first meet the person I'm working with," she said, "I like to just observe, be with them, and try to connect. There isn't always a clear reason for a referral to music therapy from the family or care staff or even the client themselves. At that early stage, I don't use a standardized assessment because I'm often not certain where we're headed. Is it to help them with a movement disorder or with their anxiety, or are they really interested in learning an instrument but happen to be blind? Did they also just lose their spouse or is a youth going through a life transition?

"It may not be clear at first whether I'm going to be needed in a counselling role or provide adaptive music education or work on rehabilitation. But that role becomes apparent as I spend time with the person and we tentatively try a song or an instrument together. When I get to know them, build a relationship, read their clinical file, and speak to other members of the interdisciplinary team or a child's parents, what I initially thought might be most beneficial can change."

I commented on how different music therapy must be from a deterministic field like pharmacy, where a dose of two hundred milligrams of a particular substance will yield a fairly predictable result.

"Music is indeed different," she agreed. "I can't predict if my flute will ring nicely to your ears. I offer it, because that's one of the tools I have to offer. I know how it has affected listeners' breathing in the past, and what kinds of memories and other responses it may elicit.

"I want to find out what music you know and like, and how to connect it to your needs and challenges and strengths.

"And you always have the option to say no or to request a song or to wave your hand to the ebb and flow of the melody. So in that sense, I invite you to play and explore with me.

"What can you tell me about play in the sense of just having fun together?" I asked, wondering if I was posing one of those simple questions for which there's no simple answer. "Of finding a musical experience pleasurable. Where does that fit into what you're trying to accomplish?"

Annette thought about this question for a moment. "Wherever there's play, wherever there is creativity, there's the potential to solve problems you can't solve by any other means. To look at a situation from a different angle." Her voice grew more animated. "And music is a form of symbolic communication that goes beyond, and sometimes deeper, than the verbal. Add in the spontaneous joy of an interaction that music can facilitate, and we're a step ahead. We can experience that joy with every client group, whether I'm working with seniors with dementia, young adults with developmental disabilities, or children with autism."

She had relaxed totally, some twinkle returning to her eyes. "Sorry. I'm getting a little enthusiastic."

Now it was my turn to think for a few moments. "Going back to what you were just saying about getting to know the person and building a relationship, do you have any quick and easy examples of what that can look like?"

"You mean in the context of assessment and the deepening of therapeutic relationships?"

"Sure, that would work."

She glanced towards a barking dog in a neighbour's yard while she began speaking. "One of my colleagues works in palliative care. Clients might ask her to play only happy songs, which, of course, she can and will do. But she may suspect their request is because they're afraid to admit to feeling sad or they're anxious about dying. So at some point, she might say, 'I notice how important this happy music is for you. What are you experiencing while you listen or sing? How does the music help you in what you are going through?'

"In this way, she opens the door to talking about sorrow and fear, and then she waits to see if the person is willing to enter into what might be an important conversation. Whether they do depends partly on the individual, but also on how safe and comfortable they feel with the therapist."

I said this was the type of illustration I sought. "Now, how about an example of a therapeutic relationship from your own work? Perhaps from long-term care?"

"Oh golly, where to begin? There's so much I could say." She drummed her fingers as she considered how to respond. Finally she said a few words about a person-centred philosophy of care. "Geriatricians, nurses and care aides, housekeepers, and recreation therapists may all work from this philosophy, and yet long-term care remains dominated in many ways by the medical model. It's such a controlled environment.

"So when I come along as the music therapist I'm very aware that I'm entering the residents' home. As much as I can in this environment, I try to give my long-term care clients a high degree of control in the way I approach them. I seek to encourage their independence and choice, and to honour their life experience.

"By the way, this approach isn't unique to music therapy. I'm happy to say that many others in health care also identify with patients, trying to create some interactive, open spaces where the patient is in the driver's seat.

"This also means that even though I'm the clinician with something to offer, I need to know when to step back and listen. Or when to leave the room. I need to know when not to challenge someone who is really hardened in their shell." Annette smiled, tilting her head as she added, "Although I might come back later and ask, 'Is this a good time for me to visit?'"

I asked whether wanting clients to participate voluntarily works as well in practice as in theory. Sometimes the realities of a workplace make it difficult to implement a cherished philosophy.

Annette said she always asks, not only whether her presence is welcome but also whether the client likes the sound or activity. She's always willing to change or substitute an activity. "In the places I've worked, music therapy was offered as a choice. Sometimes the residents had very few choices left. Just because somebody looks bored and disengaged and non-participatory, I would never assume." She explained that she's also always monitoring their body language, facial expressions, and instant reactions. "We're trained to be gentle and to be listeners and to respond to moment-to-moment needs."

※ ※ ※

Annette's parents, along with many others in the northern European community where she grew up, encouraged her passion for music. Most importantly, they shared their own enthusiasm and served as role models. When her mother was a girl, she had joined a folk singing group. Her father, who had a fondness for tenor voices, sang in a men's choir for over forty years. "Going to those concerts my dad sang in, I loved the music but didn't realize as a youngster that singing was something you could learn or study."

Annette started with some early childhood music education classes, "where I was a real rascal." Then she entered her elementary school's Orff program, which combined vocal and instrumental music on Orff instruments, drama, movement, and speech arts. The principal arranged the music for xylophones, metallophones, drums, and recorders, and toured the school's ensemble to neighbouring schools. He also taught Annette piano, after school, free of charge.

"In Grade 3, I had my first paid gigs playing recorder trios with two friends for baptisms in the local Roman Catholic church. Apparently we were very cute musicians."

The town's deep appreciation of, and commitment to, the arts came through in what Annette described next: "In Grade 5, I took up the flute. Our town had a very good, municipally subsidized community music school where the more family members you signed up, the cheaper it would become for each participant. If your parents volunteered—served on the board, for example—the costs dropped further. It was affordable even for our family. Then, a few years later, I joined the youth orchestra, having started learning the viola. I didn't get very far with the viola, but it was great fun because I could play in the string quartet and orchestra. We'd go on orchestra retreats, and I just loved it.

"I never knew how much the school cost. I'd ask, but my parents would hum and haw and sigh. They wouldn't have been able to afford ballet or tennis or horseback riding, but my parents could wrap their heads around music education. They were very supportive."

The town also had a century-long tradition of mounting a children's theatre production each summer. "For six weeks, the majority of kids in town would rehearse and then take part in perhaps two dozen performances in the afternoon and evening. It would be a fairy tale set to music, played by a live children's and youth orchestra in the pit. That was just the most wonderful experience."

Annette was immersed in music long before high school. When she reached Grade 5, she opted for the music and language stream rather than the math and science option.

Her story intrigued me because I couldn't imagine my childhood town providing so many inexpensive arts opportunities for youth. I now understood how her musical and cultural background might have made music therapy a natural career choice. But her occupation requires more than musical skills. It also requires very strong social skills. "It's one thing for a young person to learn how to get along with their peers," I said. "But in your job you have to relate well to all sorts of people. Was there anything in your upbringing that helped strengthen your people skills?"

Annette pondered this. "Well, growing up, I had really good relationships with my four grandparents. I felt very loved, and I relished listening to their stories." She slowed down. "But lots of kids have that experience, and yet find it hard to relate to people outside their immediate family and circle of friends."

After a long silence while looking up into the branches of her apple tree, she turned to me again. "My first job was delivering church newsletters every week and collecting the money once a month. I inherited this little job from my cousin. When I was gathering the money from what were mostly older people, they'd invite me in for tea. I'd admire the doilies, listen to their stories, and look at their photo albums. I had a lovely time. A route that could have taken forty-five minutes usually took two to three hours because I visited so much along the way.

"I also worked as a camp counsellor for several summers, initially with typical children and then with kids with additional support needs. Before graduating from high school, I did a practicum at a segregated school for children with developmental disabilities. It was a very good school and I learned a lot about working in the field of special education."

Although Annette's upbringing prepared her well for music studies at university, and she liked what she knew of the field, she wasn't ready to commit to it and forego other possibilities. "In my last year of high school, I really didn't know what direction I wanted to go. I attended a one-week career orientation course at the Waldorfschule in Stuttgart. We got introduced to medicine, music therapy, architecture, curative education, and teaching. I really liked what I heard about music therapy."

I asked about the concept of the Waldorfschule, and Annette explained that this type of private school follows the teachings of Rudolf Steiner and his educational and spiritual philosophy of anthroposophy. The mantra of this holistic way of learning is along the lines of engaging the child's head, heart, and hands.

I nodded as she returned to her story. "When I finished high school, I had the travel bug. A relative suggested I visit Canada, where he lived. At much the same time, the director of the music school said he could get me a Rotary scholarship to attend the Toronto conservatory of music. I didn't take him up on this offer, perhaps because I didn't think of myself as a good enough musician."

Although she was not keen about studying at that stage of her life, Annette still wanted to travel overseas, somewhere far away. "So I applied to intentional communities where families and staff lived with kids and adults with special needs. I inquired about places in Australia, South Africa, and Canada. In the summer of 1989 I ended up being invited to come to Canada for a year, to the Laurentian mountains, north of Montreal. Upon arrival, I immediately met my future husband, but that's a different story."

When Annette returned to Europe a year later, she continued to dither about where to go and what to do. She admired her older sister's choice of curative education—a Steiner concept that blends social work, music therapy, and some care aide functions in a single occupation. "I considered music therapy. I considered education. I went back and forth about those. I looked into occupational therapy. Finally I decided to go into education."

While studying at university to become a teacher, she became enamoured with homeschooling. "I got a grant to write my thesis about homeschooling in Canada. That was also a way I could keep in touch with my boyfriend." The project deepened her knowledge of some of the less savoury historical forces that shaped schooling for the masses. Having seen a way of educating children outside the school system, she completed her degree in education but chose to forego the subsequent internship required for certification as a schoolteacher. Instead she applied to the Bachelor of Music Therapy program at Capilano University in North Vancouver.

"I auditioned on the phone. Because I already had a bachelor's degree with a major in music and psychology, I met most of Cap's prerequisites in terms of first- and second-year courses. I only had to take an additional course or two in Europe to become fully eligible to start third year at Cap. I immigrated in August and began the program in September. So music therapy was the route by which I entered Canadian society."

I said I could imagine what her coursework might have been like, but I was curious about her time as an intern. "Internship can be a weird, in-between experience in some professions. A time when there's a lot of trial and error. Was it intense for you? Rewarding and valuable?"

"Some of the time, for sure. Let me see if I can recall something that was fairly positive and then something that was more challenging." She cupped her hands around her cheeks and stared into the soft hues of the approaching twilight.

She began by describing a local municipality that hired a few music therapy students for six weeks each summer to lead sing-along groups for seniors. The students rotated through the municipality's long-term care facilities, which gave the students valuable experience and freed up some of the regular staff to take vacation.

"I met an Austrian lady who was a Holocaust survivor. She was the first Jewish person I had ever met. A former musician, she took me under her wing and offered me a most gracious friendship. She taught me a lot about forgiveness. But as lovely as the experience was for me, I remained on edge because the program involved some life review and reminiscing. For somebody like her, that was easier said than done. Reminiscing can really lead you down a rabbit hole."

Next, Annette described a placement at an inner-city elementary school, saying it had been intense, a failure, and a great learning experience. She and a colleague had obtained a grant to launch an after-school music program, one which they hoped would attract a fair number of the school's Indigenous students. "As a recent immigrant, I was totally unprepared for the setting. Getting to know the families and their struggles was really meaningful, but I was naive about the history of residential schools, intergenerational suffering, and the perception of myself as a white settler. It was a place that could easily lead to burnout.

"I needed way more training than I had at the time. More training and better supervision. We also came to realize that nobody would hire us afterwards, based on this internship. My partner decided to switch into teacher training. We spent only part of the grant, returned the rest, and abandoned the project. But I think it was a good start, a brave start."

When she eventually completed her internship, the next step was to become accredited as a music therapist. "At the time, the requirement was to present a portfolio and a case study documenting my skills, knowledge, and experience. The accreditation file has since been augmented with a certification exam."

※ ※ ※

I commented that my brief browsing of a few university websites had revealed, even to a layperson, that schools varied in their approach to educating music therapists. "Yes," Annette replied. "There are half a dozen programs in Canada, and each is distinct. Some are very strong in clinical improvisation, where you really analyze your music-making. You record it and look at the chords you played with the melodies, down to the finest detail. Some are offshoots of music training. There's Concordia, with its strong creative arts focus. The program in Manitoba is offered at a faith-based institution, Canadian Mennonite University."

"Did that variety also seem to be the case in Europe?"

"I would say yes," she replied slowly. "I'd also say the field was already more mainstream. In Germany and Austria, the founding fathers seem to have been Orff, Steiner with his anthroposophy, and others who developed a fairly psychoanalytic stream. In England, there were Paul Nordoff and Clive Robbins who worked as co-therapists with individual children. The co-founder of the first Canadian program, Nancy McMaster at Capilano, had been educated under Robbins in England, and then had done her master's degree in the States at NYU."

I asked where Capilano fit into this landscape, what its distinguishing ethos had been.

"It was an interesting place," Annette said, "because it was firmly grounded in more than one cultural tradition and gave us a solid introduction to several of the theories of music therapy. The other co-founder of the program, Carolyn Kenny, was of mixed European and Indigenous heritage. This led to a strong focus on understanding both health care culture and the Indigenous roots of healing.

"There's a founding myth that Carolyn and Nancy met hitchhiking to Vancouver. The first music therapy they did, called the Children's Spontaneous Experimental Music Workshop, was out of a little minivan or Volkswagen bus. They'd show up at children's centres, or wherever they worked, barefoot and in flowing skirts. Very hippie.

"So from one side, yes, you could be barefoot, but you also had to be able to wear the language and demeanour and craft of health care professionals."

Annette sat quietly for a moment. "Because music therapy was so recent and grassroots in Canada, Cap College must have taken a big leap of faith in deciding to offer music therapy. The program taught us not to expect established positions when we graduated. Economically, Canada was changing towards the gig economy in the mid-1990s when I was a student. So we had a lot of practice with interviews, grant writing, doing unpaid work, and volunteering. We learned to be very creative in how we presented ourselves.

"Not our practicums so much but our internships were usually at places where we created a position for ourselves. Often we were the only music therapist at the site. We didn't get paid during the internship. In fact, we usually paid the music therapist who came to supervise us."

Ouch, I thought. *Most students only have tuition fees and book costs to contend with.* "In addition to the internship at the end of your program, did you get much by way of practicum experience?"

Annette started counting on her fingers. "I can recall four, each in a different setting. They were formative experiences for me, and I think for most of my classmates. It's one thing to practise in the classroom with peers. It's another thing to learn with actual clients."

I started to summarize what I understood to have been the characteristics of her time at Capilano. I got as far as cross-cultural learning and entrepreneurship in a changing health care landscape, but then found I lacked the language to succinctly describe the other concepts. Annette stepped in to help me: "We'd probably describe that as person-centred music therapy. I'd also add music improvisation skills and repertoire for different populations. Practice in several of the creative arts."

We seemed to have talked all we wanted about the various programs for becoming a music therapist. I wanted to turn the focus to some of her sessions with clients. She had previously mentioned a client who was a good example of her use of a particular type of therapy, neurologic music therapy, but our conversation had taken a different turn.

"Would this be a good time to tell me about the Mr. Sinclair you touched on earlier?" I asked. It was. His case turned out to be an example of Annette's ongoing professional education and how the field of music therapy is evolving.

"I can give you the short version, if you want," she offered, "but I think you'd benefit from the long version."

"The long version then."

"Okay, but remember that I did give you a choice." She became more serious. "Music therapy used to suffer because we could never fully explain why we were more than volunteer musicians or entertainers. Why did we deserve to be part of a medical or interdisciplinary team? That's still a struggle, especially where health care and education are carved up into rigidly bounded, professional domains. It's hard to break into.

"But people have shown time and again that there is a place for the humanistic model along with the medical model. There's a place for the spiritual, for hope, for meaning, love, and connection—all those words that don't perhaps have a place in a coding manual for insurance reimbursement.

"So this was the background in the early 2000s when the interface of music, medicine, brain plasticity, and neurology started taking off. We know so much more about these subjects than we used to. With functional MRIs, we can check what is happening. We don't have to do a spit test or questionnaire anymore, because we can hook clients up to a machine and check which regions of the brain light up. It's fascinating and impressive stuff. The training I took last year in Toronto was for me to catch up on developments in neurologic music therapy."

This was familiar territory for me. After having seen videos and skimmed books about the brain and music, I had glanced at Michael Thaut's book describing neurologic music therapy. He explained that modern music therapy is rooted in the social sciences, drawing on such overarching concepts as facilitating group association and social organization, emotional expression, symbolically representing beliefs and ideas, and supporting educational processes. Then in the early 1990s, music therapy expanded dramatically to become more scientific, driven by new research techniques for analyzing the brain. At the time of his writing, in 2014, twenty standardized clinical techniques for music therapists had been developed and more were anticipated as research continued.

Annette had travelled last year to the University of Toronto for some training in these neurological advancements. "It was impressive learning, and when I came back to the facility where I've been working for ten years, I wanted to apply it right away. You know how it sometimes is, when you learn something new that appeals to you.

"There was a resident, Mr. Sinclair, with whom I could never do anything. I had pretty much given up on him. His stroke, thirteen years ago, had left him with Broca's aphasia. This meant that while he could understand everything people said, what came out of his mouth was garbled goulash. After each meal, he'd just go back to his room and sit there, watching TV and not being very communicative. He had no interest in what I had to offer, and this situation had gone on for years.

"I thought of him when I came back from Toronto. All these neurologic therapies have a strict protocol that you follow, including an assessment of whether the person is a good candidate for a particular technique. I thought he was a good match for one and could be my guinea pig in my first attempt with melodic intonation therapy.

"With many of these techniques, the foundation is that rhythm, or music with a strong beat, will change your brain. It doesn't matter how long ago the injury happened. The brain can still change itself. If you have motor issues, rhythm will do that work. Rhythm will entrain the cortex, and that will change the motor cortex.

"Because my training had been so recent, I felt so prepared to do this right. It wasn't up to me to choose how I would engage with him. Rather, there was a technique for exactly his condition. His limited speech was his only impairment, nothing else. He would otherwise be a fully functioning person, mentally. But, of course, his stroke had also put him in a wheelchair, and he was paralyzed on the left side."

After hearing her explanation of what she wanted to try, Mr. Sinclair agreed to participate, and Annette began seeing him for a half-hour session each week. She wrote phrases on cue cards, using a simple notation system to indicate when the voice should rise and fall, and how long to hold each sound. "I knew he wouldn't get regular speech back, but I hoped he'd be able to manage a few phrases in a singsong rhythm. I wasn't trying to turn him into a singer. Just to exaggerate the cadences and pitches of regular speech in a form that he could reproduce."

She selected two dozen practical phrases, everyday statements such as "Come on in" and "I need to go to the bathroom." ("Co-o-ome / on in" and "I ne-e-e-d / to go-o-o / to the ba-a-ath / room.") Any tourist who has ever been adrift in a foreign country, overwhelmed by an unfamiliar language, appreciates the huge difference that a vocabulary of even fifty words can make—all the more if their sign language is restricted to using one forearm and wobbling their head.

"The technique was wonderful. Despite the infrequent and very limited time I could give him during those six months, the results amazed me. He was a most engaged learner, so eager to practise, and aware of his struggles—that awareness was one of the criteria why I considered him. He could evaluate his learning and his successes, which reinforced his motivation."

I asked if he had recovered enough to have a simple conversation. Annette said he had always been able to converse in the sense of responding with yes or no, or making noises. But expressing himself had been mainly a drawn-out game of twenty questions with partners whose skill in posing questions varied greatly, or laboriously using alphabet sheets to spell out words.

"It wasn't easy for him. Because one side of his body was paralyzed, his mouth and muscles pulled to the side. His damaged tongue had difficulty with pronunciation and word formation. But despite those barriers, he felt so hopeful. He became a little more outgoing. He was always ready for his session. He would readily sing with me, this man who wasn't a socializer. He so wanted to do this work, because, after over a decade, he was regaining his ability to initiate and steer some conversation."

Annette added that research confirms Mr. Sinclair's arm movements aided his partial recovery of speech. "So if you combine a rhythmically moving arm with singing, it actually helps them speak. It's not just an accidental by-product when people speak with their hands. The Italians were on to this centuries before the neuroscientists."

* * *

While Annette dashed inside to attend to one of her kids, I wandered over to look at a low, bushy pear tree on the other side of the property line. The tree was laden with small, partially ripened fruit, and it looked as though the branches of two plants had become intertwined. I only found one trunk, though, behind the irregular boxwood hedge that served as a fence. The black trampoline by the stairs into the kitchen next door might have been aging, but this fruit tree was thriving.

When Annette returned, I asked about the young adults she works with. I knew she was connected in some way to a community living association that helps individuals with developmental disabilities build meaningful lives outside institutions—these are people who sometimes also cope with physical or psychological challenges, along with intellectual ones. My interest lay in how she had come to that organization and how she ends up working with certain of their clients rather than others.

"It's a huge, very established agency," she began, "supporting about eight hundred clients in the suburbs. They have an art gallery. They have staff who play guitar at jam sessions, say at a coffee house or music night, or do other things along these lines. They wanted to add something musical that was more goal oriented, perhaps not leading to prescribed or predetermined results but that was person-centred and where progress could be observable by a supervisor.

"I got a phone call out of the blue, in August, two years ago. The people from Adult Services asked me if I could come in and talk to them about music therapy and maybe consult about how they could start something. So I said okay, this is me and here's the kind of experience I've had. I added that I had a friend who had worked for a similar agency for a decade. If they wanted, I could bring her along and she could describe what they did at her agency. So we went and had a meeting.

"Because my friend was about to move away and wasn't available to take on any new work, I suggested they could hire me instead. I was sort of between things, in any event, and ready for a change. I'd done a lot of music education and preschool work through a lovely, locally based program, and had also been teaching at an arts centre. I wanted to consolidate my work, to focus it a little more, because I was a bit worn out from driving to so many different preschools. This was an opening, so I took it and it worked out.

"They had a list of clients they had in mind, people who hadn't yet settled into a niche at the agency. Maybe music would be their thing. Sometimes I knew a lot about the person, sometimes I knew nothing about the person when I met them for the first time. I did have some understanding of this young adult population, though, so it felt like a natural fit. I didn't have any issues communicating or getting them to like me or any of those beginner issues when getting started."

Annette decided she would treat her clients as partners, as fellow musicians. "Obviously their inexperience or never having played or fine motor issues or gross motor issues or sensory difficulties presented themselves." The agency's directors seemed pleasantly surprised by how well most people responded, despite one or two who didn't want to attend or who dropped out after a couple of sessions. "Quitting is okay, because my approach is that this is a choice. You're not in rehab. This is your adulthood, and you should be able to do with it what you choose. So if music is up your alley, and I'm the one you want to walk up that alley with you, then I can offer my skills and my experience to make music with you and teach you and listen to you."

The plan called for a dozen sessions with each client and then another batch of clients would come along. "But what happened is that people don't really leave. I've had some people for two years, sometimes continually and sometimes off and on. Individuals coalesced into small groups." Youth who had just transitioned from high school into community living would amble over from their part of the building when the music began, joining the program for adults in their twenties and thirties. Then they'd return to whatever they had been doing previously.

When COVID arrived, everybody suddenly had to stay at home. Annette took three weeks off in March, thinking at first that her work had disappeared indefinitely. During that time her father died and "my kids were in the forever-spring-break that didn't end, so I needed to be home anyway."

She considered whether to go virtual and offer telehealth. "It soon became apparent that either the clients or their caregivers didn't have the technical know-how. The quality of the transmission can leave something to be desired. Also, many of them don't have their own musical instruments at home."

The clincher came when she speculated on what her clients were doing in their homes during COVID. "They usually go to their community inclusion programs three to five days a week. That is their normal social life. Some of them have aging parents. They're not meant to just sit at home and do nothing." Some had previously volunteered in the community or done little jobs on contract through the agency. "They might normally sit together and knit, or have art and music. Everybody had a different life, but all of a sudden everybody now had the same dull life sitting in isolation at home. So I decided to go mobile. I decided I'd visit them where they were, outdoors at their homes, and bring the studio with me."

Annette loaded her Honda with numerous instruments—African drums and guitars are awkward to pack. She met her clients, now always one-on-one, in their driveways and on back porches. She used a pointing stick to maintain social distance, sat downwind, wiped each instrument between clients, and generally increased safety protocols wherever she could. Some of her clients didn't fully understand the pandemic or why their usual activities had stopped, but they still bore the consequences. "For some participants, these brief sessions are one of the very few personal connections with the outside world, one of the few activities that bring purpose, joy, and levity to their daily lives."

An unexpected bonus of going mobile was that some family members and caregivers got to observe the sessions, learning how they could assist participants in bringing more music into their daily living. "That's a tremendous benefit for everybody in the home."

The energy propelling our discussion of clients with developmental disabilities seemed to be dissipating. We sat in companionable silence for a while. "Tell me a bit now," I suggested, "about your work with people at the other end of the age spectrum, with seniors."

"Which seniors? I've worked in seven or eight long-term care facilities over the years. Some were more supported or independent living, where residents still had their wits and were ambulatory. Then there were a couple of extended-care places with full nursing support. I even have some experience in special care with dementia patients, where the units are locked."

"How about the extreme case, with special care?"

"Okay. I've been at this long enough to have seen how philosophies of care have changed over the years. "Gentlecare" was all the rage in the nineties. Then I saw the Eden philosophy of eldercare and witnessed some attempts to make the facilities seem less institutional. They'd bring in pets and kids and music and community and gardening. Give everyone something to do. People and pets to interact with. Jobs to do, with roles and responsibilities.

"Anyhow, one of my favourite people was a lady who, due to advanced dementia, had lost most her language. She had a very supportive husband, who adored her and would bring her to my groups. He stayed because he had only her. She was his entire social network.

"This couple had been fond of music, attending concerts and familiar with all the easy classics. One day this woman's husband took a set of my rhythm sticks and gently placed them in her hands. He put his hands over hers and guided them to show her how to strike them, and rub them together, to make various sounds. Well, she twigged on to this and, to everyone's surprise, became quite a rhythmic participant. She'd never done this before, but she'd bah-da-dum, bah-da-dum, bah-da-dum-dum-dum while I accompanied her on the piano. Or I might play a part and she would play the next part. We'd pass it back and forth as I played tango, Mexican, or classical. Through this medium, an almost comatose person became extremely responsive and communicative. Fully engaged and evidently pleased with herself. Proud husband, amazed group."

I asked, "To what extent did you see the husband as your client as well? He was clearly benefiting, but you hadn't been hired to look after his needs. Yet if he's doing better, I would think this trickles over into how he cares for his wife."

"Yeah, yeah, it was helping him too. In long-term care, it's often like that. The tragedy during COVID is that all the spouses and families are shut out. It's not just the residents who receive care. It's the spouses too.

"I sometimes take the opportunity in my groups to make these relationships the topic of a discussion. We might talk about sending somebody into care, or about being the one who now lives alone in the community or has to downsize the house and move. Or maybe they don't want to accept that their spouse is dying or that they need to connect with the Alzheimer Society. All of a sudden, there are three or four couples, one a resident and one a visitor, joining the conversation. The visitor might get a sandwich and soup because they don't know how to cook very well—that's provided sort of under the table. So it's not just music therapy: it's social work too. Want it or not, you're part of the community and you have to look after people."

"You're starting to tug at my heartstrings," I said.

"Good," Annette replied. "Here's another story that I hope will resonate with you.

"When I was just starting out, I met a Hungarian immigrant at a care home who had no family at all. She was very grumpy and very unhappy—those are the best people because they usually have big reasons why they're like that. Sometimes they let you enter their space and share with you about their existence, and they let you in some tiny way be a witness to what they've gone through. I try to just listen, not fix it, although that tends to be something I want to do.

"One of her gripes was the food because none of her favourites from her youth were ever served. She had nobody to speak Hungarian with, nothing to connect her to her culture. So I decided to research some Hungarian folk music, a cumbersome process back in those pre-Internet days. I'd usually set aside one Saturday a month to do research and photocopying in the music collection at the main branch of the public library.

"As I began learning those songs and bringing them to her, she became my teacher. She corrected my pronunciation and helped me get the mood right. We sang songs together, and she would chuckle at my mistakes. Eventually she came to trust me enough to admit that she was intensely homesick.

"Now I had reached a stage where it's hard to know where my role should end, what my boundaries should be. I had told her my parents came from the same corner of the world, and we agreed that those in the Austro-Hungarian Empire had enjoyed way better food than countries with a British heritage. It was probably well beyond what I should have done, but I dug out a strudel recipe and I baked her some strudel. We reminisced over our shared cultural heritage as we nibbled our way through the mid-afternoon.

"My point is that music connects. It loosens the emotions and breaks down the barriers. People perceive it as a gift. Seniors are an appreciative bunch anyway. And they're good teachers. They're wise, they're experienced, they know a lot of stuff. Yet they may have nobody to share it with. So sometimes as a music therapist, you take on the role of a student and give long-term care residents the chance to teach and share. This matters, because a lot of life in long-term care is a drag—uncomfortable, unpleasant, and forced."

Annette seemed to anticipate some of the thoughts that were forming in my mind. "Of course, those types of stories are rare because they're so labour intensive. With limited time, I'm often looking for ways that I can do things in groups or serve as a catalyst to launch something that is partially self-sustaining."

"A catalyst?" I asked. "I'm having a hard time picturing what that might look like."

"Well, one quick and easy example is when I organize a big group of wheelchair dancing."

"Wheelchair dancing? You're confusing me even more."

"A group of volunteers, perhaps a school group, comes in so that everybody has a one-on-one helper. I've had as many as thirty or forty wheelchairs, parading through the dining room and hallways, doing our version of folk dancing with either live or recorded music. And certainly with lots of raucous singing."

"Wild. I'm sure the managers love the chaos you cause."

"I'm sure they do. Staff need a little shake-up once in a while, too, along with the residents."

She became more reflective. "Single men are hard to deal with in long-term care, especially when they're younger and they've had a stroke, or a progressive condition, and their quality of life is poor. At one time in a care facility where I worked, there were quite a few of them, mainly on the same floor. Several had large music collections. All they did was sit in their room asking the staff or caregiver to change their records or CDs for them, if they weren't able to do it themselves. They'd listen, often with the volume too loud. We'd have to ask them to turn it down, especially if they were listening to rock while we were singing "You Are My Sunshine" in a nearby lounge. They had the distinct feeling they didn't fit in, and they were right.

"Finally it dawned on me that these men had something they could share with each other. They already had all the knowledge and resources in their music collections, but they couldn't get it together themselves. They needed somebody to set something up and assemble them. So I decided to be the facilitator and organize a disc night. It became a regular activity, and I was gradually able to step back and let the residents share what they were already competent and knowledgeable about. Once again, it was as much about the social connections as the music itself."

Annette might have been talking about social connection, but money was circling through my mind. Sometimes music therapy is an expenditure, a short-term boost like a meal at a good restaurant that provides temporary pleasure, good memories, but few lingering benefits. At other times it's an investment stretching into the future, perhaps lessening or delaying the need for other supports. I recounted a story I had seen in a book about people with terminal illness.

"The couple was elderly and had been married for over half a century," I said. "It was a troubled marriage, with the couple's interactions often angry and resentful when others weren't around to witness them squabbling. The wife felt unhappy and unappreciated by her husband. The husband, in turn, felt dominated by his wife, whose version of caring for him hampered him in even expressing an opinion. And now they were in long-term care.

"A music therapist persuaded them to try playing a keyboard together. Neither knew the instrument, so they were mutually vulnerable. He sat on the bench to her left, in order to play the bass line. She played the treble. As they made their faltering start, each encouraged the other. The author wrote about the dynamic being one of balanced communication often infused with humour. The couple became partners again.

"No big deal, I suppose. A temporary experience. And yet, I couldn't help wondering whether when one of them passes, the survivor might be a little less inclined to remorse about having been a less-than-perfect spouse in their latter years. He or she could think back to their keyboard experience and remember a time of mutuality and joy. Perhaps this would soften the grieving process and reduce the outside support that might be needed during those months or years."

"Maybe," said Annette. "I'd like to think so, and it's certainly possible. But you never know. Sometimes you're indeed investing in the future, but sometimes you're just helping somebody cope with the present. That's always the case with palliative patients, although their loved ones might benefit in the future.

"Last year," Annette continued, "I met a lady in a care home who had decided to die. She was totally with it cognitively but she was frail. Her only relative, a great-granddaughter or something, lived faraway in California, and she felt she had no reason to live anymore.

"It wasn't my place to convince her otherwise, so I didn't express doubt or criticize her. But I wanted to check if there was a smidgen of willingness to engage. I always feel that as long as people are willing to engage, and don't tell me to leave the room straight away, then it's worth trying.

"It's an openness that I'm looking for. Perhaps we're trained in this. It's also a basic conviction of mine that there's usually something in most people's lives that holds them to life and keeps them breathing. This lady was a tough one because she was very convinced that she had done it all. After I attempted to visit her a few times over a span of three or four weeks, she came to recognize me and would say, 'Nope, I don't need you. Leave me alone.'

"One day, I asked again, 'Could I just sit with you? I won't say anything.' This time, to my surprise, she agreed. The following time, I said, 'You know, my first language is the same as yours.' This led to a little conversation that I think we both enjoyed. But she remained as determined as ever, and by now was refusing all food and drink. It was amazing how long she lived without water, probably ten days or so, with just sort of sponging.

"Eventually she allowed me to hum a lullaby to her. She didn't want words. As the end approached, I said, 'Now, I'm going to put my hand on your bedside. If your finger touches mine, that will mean yes. If you don't touch, that will mean no.' She sought my hand, and I did what I said I would, namely to hum a lullaby. She held my hand until I finished. Then when she let go, that was my signal to stop."

* * *

Annette sighed. "That brings me to our precarious work situation. Music therapy is *still* not considered an essential service in many places. So we spend a lot of time explaining and trying to convince funders and medical personnel of what we have to offer, speaking their language rather than our own.

"There have been times when there wasn't enough work or I wanted a certain kind of work or I was disappointed that the world isn't ready for us. I periodically toy with leaving the field, not because I don't like it but because I'm tired of not feeling recognized, of having to defend, once again, why we're doing what we're doing or why we deserve to be properly paid and have job security." She smiled ruefully. "But I always come back to it. The next time a job offer comes up, I totally jump at it. I've gained experience working from cradle to grave. It's never boring.

"But it is precarious. Many of us, myself included, work on contracts. I used to have two long-term care contracts, but I let one of them go last fall. My eleven-year contract, they just closed the door to music therapy at the end of March, saying I could come back when COVID is over.

"This COVID thing is so frustrating because I've worked through flu outbreaks in the past, wearing full personal protective equipment. Those could last for three or four weeks. The seniors were in dire straits, stuck in their rooms and getting their meals delivered, becoming very bored, and feeling very isolated. But I was able to provide service. I would take my instruments down the hallway, playing at a distance, being careful where I touched and how I breathed. So to now be told to stay home because it's too dangerous feels like a slap in the face. But, being on contract, it's far easier to dispose of me than salaried employees. I think COVID has been a pretty shocking experience for many of us."

I thought back to Annette's description of her training and its emphasis on being entrepreneurial, of carving a niche for oneself in the workplace. I asked her how frontline staff view her, wondering to what extent they embrace her as part of the team.

"Those care aides," she said, "have an extremely high workload. They need to be very task oriented to get it all done. They usually work short-staffed. People are heavy, and they often need two aides for lifting, perhaps using equipment. And who wants to stare a bowel movement in the face every couple of hours? It's not always a pleasant job. Yet, there are countless care aides who manage to make somebody absolutely yummy smelling and beautifully dressed and looking their best for the day ahead. They do this every day, day after day.

"But then when they're done with their tasks, and the people are fed, they need to put the residents somewhere. That's when the non-hospital part of living in residential care begins. That's where recreation and music therapy are extremely important.

"Care homes used to have more community. The doors weren't quite so closed. Now the flu season often shuts out the community entirely for several months in the winter. It used to be that there were many more visits from Girl Guides and Boy Scouts, and preschools and day cares, and high school performers coming in. There were intergenerational programs. Maybe some facilities are still strong in that. Some definitely aren't.

"I feel you need staff who look after what makes a person's life interesting and meaningful and fun, and allows everyone to experience something worthwhile. It's not just what's on the calendar and scheduled from ten to eleven. It's also all the little interactions, the transitions from one activity to another, the approach. It's seeing somebody as a full person, not just as a bum to be wiped.

"Music therapists have a lot of training in that regard. How to defuse aggressive outbursts. How to soothe somebody when they have a meltdown or are sad or grieving. Unfortunately, care aides and nurses don't always have the time. But we're there. We should be giving that kind of support.

"Just because we're music therapists doesn't mean I always have to walk around with my guitar strung to my back. It also means that I can sit silently at somebody's bedside. I can do palliative care. I can talk with families. I can provide a connection between the spouses, perhaps when one spouse lives in an assisted wing and the other lives in full care. Or when somebody returns from hospital, there's somebody there to provide comfort and lower their anxiety and stress.

"As a member of the care team, I've taken people to the washroom. I've fed people. I took education on assessing swallowing and making sure people sit upright. That's just fine by me. That doesn't mean I take away anybody's job. It just means that the nurse could also sing a song, and the care aide, if they have twenty minutes, could also bring out a guitar. The roles don't have to be so strict.

"Because music, and music therapy by extension, is a choice, somebody can tell me to shut up but not go away. They may need me as a person, not as a songstress. I listen to their story, knowing that when they pass away, I might be the one telling it at their celebration of life. Many facilities don't have pastoral care on staff—maybe just a few volunteers, with varying amounts of time and skill to offer—so sometimes it's the music therapist who facilitates the memorial service. I've been invited numerous times to play a person's favourite songs at their funeral because the family knew me from the care facility."

Annette's comments prompted me to recall the story about the rewritten lyrics that Amy had heard at the hospice tea, and how much my horizons had broadened about music therapy since my fateful conversation with her.

"I have another question," I said, "about your challenging work situation. It's the trend of putting headphones on patients with dementia and playing favourite tunes from their youth. There seem to be some positive results from this approach, yet it feels a bit like an attempt to automate your role, perhaps an attempt to make you redundant. What are your thoughts about this?" I held my breath because I didn't know whether Annette would interpret this as an innocent question or a loaded one that might unleash a torrent.

I received a measured response: "My feelings are mixed because canned music is both positive and negative for vulnerable populations.

"We know that favourite music, especially for people with dementia, raises the heart rate. It also helps us relax. It triggers the right hormones and can be a stress release. If you're in an unfamiliar environment, familiar music will help put you at ease. It releases memories that would otherwise not be accessible. That's very clear, and was clear before they came up with the iPod.

"It can be lovely, for example, for spouses to listen together in a lounge with two headphones and a splicer. They do this together, listening to the same music. It's joined attention. It's sharing. It's beautiful.

"In long-term care, which is so hospital-medical oriented and where there is so much background noise, the environment can distract from being able to concentrate or having a thought. So wearing headphones cuts down on the background noise and lets you focus on the music better. That is true.

"However, what about that Holocaust survivor I told you about? Suppose someone happened to put on some German music. When she's had enough, is she capable of taking the headphones off? What memories are being triggered? Have they just created a perfect storm for her, maybe?

"When I'm working with a client, I'm always observing and making sure they can deal with the music or the activity. I watch the breathing, I watch for tension in the face or in the body, whether the movements are jerky or rhythmic. Are they trying to play along? Are they moving away from me? Are they closing their eyes because they're listening or overstimulated? That's a big difference between what I do and using a device."

* * *

The right team had handily won the hockey game, the shadows were lengthening, and our talk needed to draw to a close. "You've been generous, spending far more time with me than I expected. Thanks," I said. "By way of a wrap-up, let me ask what keeps you going? Is it the music itself, and being able to share and play with it in so many ways, or is there something else?"

Annette looked befuddled as she processed my question. "Many things, I guess." Her next words sounded carefully chosen. "What has inspired me, right from the beginning, are the clients. Just because of my role, of the angle I present to them, people often open up to me in a way that perhaps they wouldn't with a different caregiver.

"If there's nothing they want to share, then I can give them the gift of music. Sometimes I have to play randomly because I'm stuck about what to do in a given moment, but usually there's a touch point of connection that will lead us down a certain road. Especially with seniors, but also with patients at the cancer agency or youth at risk or prisoners in jail or people with addictions—not that I've worked in all those fields—music seems to be something that we can hold in common. It touches us all, and there's a togetherness, a sharing that's unique to the field of music. Our shared humanity.

"I've met so many people, so many individuals. I love listening to their stories, being this private little historian for a while. Music may trigger a memory or reinforce someone's belief in themselves, give them hope, or make them move or enable them to have fun within a body that is otherwise very limited. I've always felt very privileged to be able to meet all these people."

"I wouldn't have been able to articulate that," I commented, "but now that you've said it out loud, it seems obvious. Relationships and sharing were themes in so much of what you talked about."

"Yes, that's true," Annette said. "Everyone once in a while when I'm in a care home I feel like I'm a preteen again, back with the little old ladies and their teacups and doilies, back when I was delivering my church newsletters. It's more of a spontaneous love for the other and a delight to be together and a recognition that we each have something that is darling to the other.

"And that sharing and delight manage to co-exist with some very practical considerations. I'm constantly assessing, developing new short-term objectives towards a long-term goal, and always looking for ways to make improvements. If I'm dealing with life-threatening or progressive diseases, then I'm trying to maintain or slow down the decline. Hang on to the plateau a little longer. For therapists who work in rehab, they're trying to elevate the level of functioning."

As I started my leave-taking, and Annette was walking with me to my car, she asked if she had been sufficiently clear that she sought to avoid becoming the centre of attention in her work. "It's never my performance or me being the famous teacher. It's always about the client, whether it's an autistic person drumming to learn control and interaction or a child singing and dancing to express themselves. One of the concepts I like is the notion that the music is actually a co-therapist.

"We music therapists are not sound healers. I'm not sure we especially consider ourselves as western-trained healers. But we do acknowledge all the elements of music, whether it's on a cellular level that makes your muscles move or an emotional one that's linked to the timbre of an instrument or a long-term memory. In this sense, the music is that third member in the relationship. I'm not the star."

Traffic was light that evening, and the route familiar, so driving home required little concentration. I pondered Annette's emphasis that music in her work is always a choice. "I never want to force anybody to have me," she had said on a couple of occasions. "If I'm too loud or don't do something the way you like, just tell me. If that's not what you need, then I understand." My own work life had been rather different: I occasionally had to write reports containing unwelcome information that my readers would have preferred to ignore or discard. They would have loved the option of pushing me away.

Music therapy's advantage is that music is usually welcome and motivating. It's something people are curious about, something that is pain free. I flipped through my notes when I arrived home.

Her comments weren't entirely what I remembered, in that I had forgotten she said she sometimes has to exercise a little overt or covert persuasion at first.

She also said that although music therapy differs from entertainment, people may nevertheless think music is only for when they're in a good mood, for when they're doing well. "Then I explain that music therapy is different. You can benefit from it when you're in a crabby mood or in pain—especially when you're in pain. So if you're in a bad headspace, whether you're at the cancer agency, or you're a survivor of abuse, or you're moping in residential care, let's see if a little carefully chosen music can help you gain a foothold to a better frame of mind."

ANTONIO

Antonio shifted his practice some years ago from seniors in long-term care to a younger adult population with concurrent disorders: "a diagnosed mental illness combined with addiction," he explained. "Heavy-duty stuff. The program at this place is residential, with clients often staying for upwards of half a year. It's government funded, so it's not luxurious, but the staffing is reasonably comprehensive as these things go."

My cousin had introduced me to Antonio during a quick trip I made to the Prairies. To my surprise and delight, not only was he willing to show me his workplace but our schedules also permitted this to happen.

He led me into the music studio—definitely not a bland, institutional venue—in the large health and social services facility where he works part-time. The overhead fluorescent fixtures in the windowless room were off; instead, a couple of floor lamps provided subdued, atmospheric lighting. The equipment was mainly electronic and, to my eye, sophisticated. Where were the tambourines, African drums, and shakers that I associate with music therapy? Instead, four or five electric guitars hung on a wall, with two acoustic ones propped in stands on the floor. A black electronic drum set filled a corner, leaving ample room for a professional-grade keyboard in front of the guitars. I glanced at what seemed to be a mixer or soundboard on a workbench attached to the opposite wall, along with some computers.

My rubbernecking was hardly subtle. "We're pretty well equipped," he acknowledged as he gave me a moment to take it all in. "It's taken a long time to assemble, though. Some donations, but mainly funded from a small annual budget. The latest addition is that projector." He pointed to a white machine that I guessed cost several hundred dollars.

After draping my jacket over the back of an upholstered vinyl armchair—the only aspect of the studio that shouted institutional—I settled into the seat and turned my attention back to Antonio. "How was it that you became a music therapist?"

He leaned forward, and his salt and pepper goatee darkened under the shift in lighting. "You may not be stunned to learn that I took piano lessons and music theory as a kid. Thinking I'd maybe become a school music teacher, I started off studying education at university. Not a good fit, so I quickly switched into a Bachelor of Music program, majoring in composition. I liked the creativity. But after graduation I ended up giving private piano and theory lessons—okay, at best, and not a career path I wanted to pursue."

During his university summers, Antonio had worked in his hometown hospital, running the switchboard and doing some admitting. "I liked that setting," he said. "I was aware of music therapy from books I had stumbled upon in the music library while I was a student. I started speculating whether that occupation might be a good marriage for me of a hospital setting and music."

"Music therapy wasn't mentioned in your music program?"

"No, nobody talked about it. The field wasn't as well known then."

So Antonio returned to school. His first few jobs as a newly minted music therapist were in geriatrics. "But I always wanted to do more in-depth work than I felt I could in nursing homes," he said. "Use more counselling skills. When this position with concurrent disorders became available, the hours were the same as what I was working at one of my long-term care homes. That made it feasible to switch into this line of work a decade ago. It's been wonderful."

"You mentioned counselling skills. Would you have been able to work with this challenging population as a fresh grad, or would you have needed more training and experience?"

Both, it seemed, were true. "When I trained in music therapy, none of us would have had the necessary skills without having matured and gained life experience. Students who are graduating now are able to pop into this type of work. There's more meat to the training now." Nevertheless, a master's degree in counselling psychology remains a popular choice for music therapists wanting to augment their skills.

***

"I'm really out of my element here," I said, stating the obvious. "Schizophrenia, borderline personality disorder, bipolar disorder. Opioid addiction, problem gambling. These just haven't been part of my experience, not even second- or thirdhand, so I can't begin to guess what your workweek looks like. Could you give an overview for somebody who has led a very sheltered life?"

"So neither have you experienced any bouts of homelessness, poor dental care, or sexual abuse?"

"No."

"Then count your blessings. Detoxing our clients is just the start of their recovery, and of learning ways to cope with what might be lifelong challenges. Music therapy is one piece of a much bigger treatment effort, but it's a piece that I think you'll be able to relate to."

Antonio had a knack for putting me at ease. He started by telling me that clients may choose to come to the centre, assuming they meet the eligibility criteria. Although such stays are voluntary, once they enter, they could be locked down for a month or two before they earn passes and get more freedom. It's not a decision to be made lightly.

I nodded in comprehension.

"It's surprising how often music therapy provides the buy-in for treatment. Potential and new clients get toured around. Sometimes they walk in here and their mouths hang open. 'Oh, there's a recording studio. Wow, look at all the guitars,' they say. It seems like a simple thing, but for people with at least one serious diagnosis, like antisocial personality disorder, plus addiction and maybe cognitive impairment from drug use, music is familiar and more accessible than heavy talk-based groups.

"And then, once they're in residence, I like taking clients off the unit because the studio is normalizing. It can be dispiriting to be locked in an assessment unit until you earn passes and such."

I asked about the centre's involuntary clients. "How do they come to be here?"

"Sometimes the court sends them because their doctors have certified them as unable to make healthy decisions for themselves. Those certifications come up for review by a panel every two or three months. Others avoid jail by opting for treatment instead."

"That's quite the population you're working with. How do you go about it?"

"We're group based here, although I do see some people individually by referral. I'm seeing three people one-to-one right now, which is one more than I really should, being part-time. That number ebbs and flows.

"The groups usually meet once a week for an hour, or thirty minutes when we're in the assessment unit. In an ideal world, six clients are plenty. Other groups at the centre are held in the auditorium, where they sit in rows like in a movie theatre. I prefer everyone being able to see each other, making it easier for clients to talk and ask questions among themselves. I don't like to be the sole leader in the room, with everyone talking only to me or with me imparting all the information.

"I probably spend sixty percent of my time in programs, with the remainder of my time spent on the bureaucratic and follow-up activities. I usually do three to four programs a day. Depending on the types of programs, that can be plenty."

"Tell me about the background, administrative stuff," I interjected. Seeing his look of surprise, I explained that I used to be a bureaucrat. "I appreciate how important the behind-the-scenes activity can be for helping things work well." Then I flustered him by asking about charting, perhaps the one and only time anybody outside his workplace would care about it.

"It varies" was his first, and not very helpful, response.

"So tell me how it varies."

"It can be as simple as a group entry to say that these people attended such and such a group, and this is what the group is about. If I have more specific details to share, then I'll make an individual entry in a SOAP format."

"SOAP?"

He hung his head and raised his shoulders, as he explained the acronym: subjective, objective, assessment, and plan. "I usually err on the side of writing more—that's my style. I'm careful, though, about how much I disclose, questioning whether all staff need to know certain details. It's not a tell-all so much as noting areas of concern."

"And do you attend case conferences?"

"Rounds are integral. I find out who is new and what's going on with them. I get to learn about different sides of the clients, especially in the assessment unit where everybody initially stays. With those who have been here for a while, I can comment on what I've observed of them."

"And what sorts of preparation do you have to do each week?"

Some of what Antonio recounted resembles the scheduling any leader has to do. "I plan what we're going to do for a grounding experience or creative arts–wise. Creative arts could be dance or movement, like a power pose. We might do a life line, where you draw a timeline on paper and add all the significant events of your childhood. With songs, there could be lyric analysis."

I was a little surprised to learn that he also teaches during some sessions. "Staff know about the importance of family and personal histories, about trauma and recovery, but simply having experienced these doesn't mean the clients somehow magically understand what has happened to them. So sometimes I'll show a couple of PowerPoint slides with talking points that I've tailored to the group. The slides might only take a few minutes to prepare, but I'm running a variety of groups each week."

The slides also prove helpful when a newcomer joins a group midstream. "Sometimes I meet individually with newcomers and go over the slides about, say, adverse childhood theory and how that connects with their experience and their scores on their assessment test. It's a good introduction because we both get to talk. I find out about them, and they get to know me. Then when they come to the group, they're not just jumping in cold or I'm not having to rush them through a quick review."

At the beginning, very few clients can manage their calendar independently. "I print up invitations to put on their doors, because so many need prompts. I'm fortunate to have an intern who posts the reminder on all the doors the day before. This really keeps the numbers up and maintains the group's continuity. As time passes, these reminders become less important."

If clients don't show up, Antonio generally looks for them later. "If they did come but were new, I'll also likely seek them out and ask how the session was for them, and how they are feeling now. It takes a lot of time."

* * *

"How old was this guy? I thought you said mid-twenties, but that kind of sounds like the behaviour of a young teen."

Antonio hinted that was the point of the story. "A psychologist would say Gobind presented as regressed in age. He also had an inflated sense of ego and was overly eager to step up to the microphone. His lyrics were grandiose and involved sexual jokes and gratuitous violence, emulating what he described as the essence of rap.

"Now before you judge him too harshly, Bob, let me tell you that Gobind was still grieving his father's death a decade earlier. He found his mother to be particularly overbearing, and reported passive suicidal thoughts in response to her." At this point in his stay, the centre's staff had hypothesized that he was compensating for his sense of worthlessness—a compensation amplified by psychotic features of grandiosity—by describing himself as the king and aspiring to become a kickboxing champion. "Part of my task was to help him process his feelings of depression and loss after his father's death and to cope more effectively with his enmeshed and dysfunctional family."

I drew in my breath. "How do you even start doing something like that?"

"Well, in this case, the song he wrote was entitled "Why I Started Drugs." I simply asked him to help me understand the connection between the lyrics and why he began using substances. My immediate objective was to get him to reflect on how he might mask his own thoughts and feelings by emulating the personas of rappers."

"Sorry, but I'm circling back to what you said a moment ago. I can't let it go. Whatever the underlying causes, Gobind was incredibly rude to that woman. She must have felt terrible."

"Of course. But rather than scold the guys about their misogyny, my approach is to calmly let them know that certain behaviour isn't okay, and that part of recovery is exploring how to have healthy, respectful relationships with ourselves and others." He paused. "Do I sound like a therapist or what? In any event, I turn the issue back to them by asking them to take some responsibility, suggesting they perhaps start by brainstorming ways of making amends."

"And did that work with Gobind?"

"I don't know. A short while later he got himself into trouble elsewhere in the centre and had to leave. Relapses are a normal part of the reality I deal with. He may resurface in the future, but right now I have no idea where he is or how he's doing."

✲ ✲ ✲

Clients don't have to participate in music therapy groups. However, if they do choose to attend, they're normally expected to make a decent effort to participate. "Sometimes they'll come, but just want to watch. I'll usually let them, especially the first time they ask. Sometimes they're nervous or dealing with other issues. I've found that if I'm too pushy, they might not come back at all, so it's a fine balance.

"But if they return the following week and still only want to observe, I'll tell them they need to do a little more than that. They have to work in some way on their mental health. Plus, I remind them that participation will help them earn a voucher."

The vouchers are a little reward system, used throughout the centre, which clients can redeem for deodorant, a toothbrush, or other necessities. It's a tangible way of encouraging them and providing concrete evidence that they are indeed making progress, however incrementally.

A different problem occurs when clients enjoy a group so much, or benefit sufficiently, that they don't want to leave. Newcomers arrive, and the size of the group creeps up to ten. "Then I consider starting a second group, but complications can arise if some clients want to alternate between groups, or even attend both groups."

Fundamentally, Antonio's role is to assist clients in becoming active meaning-makers and agents in their health. It's frequently about creating starting points for more in-depth conversations. Song lyrics, for example, can help clients relate to themselves more profoundly than in traditional talk therapy, accessing memories and disclosing thoughts and emotions they might normally keep buried. Not always, of course, but often enough.

"This health promotion goal sounds all warm and fuzzy," I commented. "But let's face it, one of your more popular groups writes and records rap. Not always the most wholesome of musical genres. How do you avoid reinforcing outlooks you're trying to change in that group?"

Antonio smiled broadly and stretched out in his chair, clasping his hands behind his head and gazing upwards. "Yeah, I get a bit of pushback about that group. Quite a bit, sometimes, when people first hear about it. But I usually win the sceptics over. The fact is that rap offers immediate access to topics like oppression, social justice, feminism, and empowerment."

"Come again?"

"Well, on one occasion, an all-male group decided to write about women and drugs, and their perceptions of the connection between the two. Our follow-up discussion centred on how the clients chose female partners who also use substances. And from there, it's a short leap into talking about empowerment or feminism or any number of topics.

"Not everybody steps forward to join this group. Sometimes we have to nudge clients we think would benefit from it. Once there, participants are pretty supportive of each other. It's common to hear applause after a client's recording. We cover everything from song title and theme selection, beat selection, and lyric writing through to recording each client's track, listening to the collective rap, and post-recording processing."

Our conversation slowed, and I used the lull to decide what else I wanted to learn about groups. "What's your favourite group?" rose to the top of my list. "At the moment or in the past, if you happen to be in bleak stretch right now."

"Adverse childhood experiences" was his immediate response. The group's origins lay in a video on the topic by a local physician that was accompanied by a ten-item questionnaire that viewers were asked to complete about their own childhoods. "Most scored really high on it, which is to say they got off to a rotten start in life. It was such a good film, but we didn't have anything in our programming that would allow us to directly continue with the topic. So I proposed starting a group."

A committee approves all new groups. Antonio presented research showing that people may need more than talk therapy to recover from traumatic or prolonged adverse experiences. Several studies have documented how victims experiencing stress in the present can perceive it as a return of the original trauma and thus revert to their earlier, dysfunctional behaviour. Drawing on what is known as attachment theory and on emerging findings in repeat theory, Antonio proposed using music and the creative arts as a vehicle for addressing this type of emotional reaction. The committee agreed.

"When I started the group, I naively thought we'd just go through each item on the questionnaire, a topic each week. But there are lots more issues than appear on the questionnaire. Clients whose parents were addicts, for example. There's a good literature about adverse childhood, but nothing published about group therapy for it. So we're pioneers.

"I love the group," he concluded. "The clients are doing really well."

Antonio's approach runs a little contrary to the widely accepted philosophy about trauma-informed practice at many recovery centres. This approach explicitly acknowledges traumatic pasts and teaches clients coping techniques to navigate them. "My criticism of it," he said as he tented his fingers, "is that it often doesn't include talking about the actual event. It's akin to getting whiplash in a car accident and having your symptoms treated, but nobody asks you what happened. They don't want you to say you were in a car accident. They just say, 'Oh, your neck hurts. Let's treat that.'

"The emerging consensus among trauma practitioners is that if you get in there as soon as clients are stable enough, and work on the root of it—carefully, so they're not going to relapse or become more traumatized—you can actually help them get better mental health. So I feel like I walk a fine line because my preference is to break the silence, the taboos, but to do so cautiously and carefully with group members."

Antonio's phone chirped to indicate a text message had arrived. He apologized for having to read it. A mere ten seconds later, he slid the phone back into his pocket.

I asked how COVID had affected his work.

"Devastating," he replied. "We've been told not to use microphones. No droplets or spittle. Nothing that involves recording is happening. I can't hand out instruments. My colleague is still doing a singalong—the songbook is full of songs about hopefulness and fun and recovery—but I don't feel safe singing at the moment.

"I did a lot of fluffy things at the beginning of the pandemic, like showing documentaries about the stories of great bands. Name that tune. A relaxation group that wasn't really needed. Anything that would minimize contact and keep numbers small. When we developed a better sense of the virus, I was able to reintroduce more substantive material."

"What would be an example of substantive work that's still pandemic appropriate?"

He thought for a moment and then mentioned some songwriting on the assessment unit. "I present a topic like, 'Why I want to quit substances,' or a song title like, 'A year from now.' Then after handing out blank papers, I wait to see how they handle the theme and what they write about. I'm interested in their ability to follow a topic, but also in what comes out. It gives you a place to work from. You can develop awareness from there, asking questions about the lyrics.

"They're having fun at the same time as they write. I might look disengaged, but all sorts of thoughts are running through my mind. Can they guide their writing towards a complete song, and where does the story go? What's the chorus—or what they call a hook nowadays?

"'What,' I might say at some point, 'if we worked on an album?' Some get stoked about that idea, having visions of fame, but it's actually hard for them. It's a good project that requires them to complete an extended task. They learn how to use the software; they learn about editing. Lots of lyrics discussion."

✳ ✳ ✳

I now wanted to explore a different aspect of groups, beyond their format and subject matter. "So besides client engagement and some *aha* moments where they gain a bit of insight, what else happens when a session goes well? And what does it look like when a group falls flat?"

His first answer came quickly. "Sometimes they come right out and say it was good." He shrugged as he added, "And they leave in one piece."

I laughed at that one but then realized it might not be a flippant comment with this clientele.

"There's a sense of group cohesion." His words were coming less rapidly now. "They feel supported not just by staff but by each other."

"I imagine that can really vary, depending on the personalities involved?"

"Oh yes, it certainly can. That's why it takes some skill to ensure things don't go sideways. But I try to keep groups organic so that when the unexpected emerges, I can go with the flow and adapt the plan for that day. And still find benefit, of course. It's not, 'Do whatever you want today. Just be happy.'"

"Are you willing to fess up to what happens when groups don't go so well?"

"Sure. I couldn't work with this population if I was uncomfortable talking about screw-ups and what are euphemistically called 'opportunities for learning.'

"Sometimes it's as simple as a bad setting, like having to meet in the TV room. People are wanting to watch television, but I'm clearing out the room and asking who wants to stay for the group. The doors can't be closed, so other clients can wander by and linger. How do you foster cohesion and psychological safety in those circumstances?

"And as you mentioned earlier, having one challenging personality, such as someone who wants to control the session, or is needy and anxious, can be tough. I hardly ever kick anyone out, though. I set limits, but I usually look for ways for everyone to manage what's going on. Maybe it's as basic as letting the person pace for a while. I watch the other clients' reactions to that client. I'm very aware that these tough moments can also be teachable ones. Unexpected opportunities to make a big impact."

Antonio reiterated that he can be firm and give direct feedback when the rules of the facility, or of the client's individualized health plan, have been violated. But he's also mindful that clients are dealing with numerous mental and life issues or may be freshly arrived at the centre and not yet fully assessed and acclimatized to it. "I'm frequently strict, but I don't get mad." He paused. "Or if I do, I don't show it. You have to maintain a sense of calm for the group, just to keep things together."

Maybe it was because of what he wasn't saying, of his silence about the irritation and disappointment he must frequently feel, that I told him he seemed committed to his clients well beyond what his job might require. He looked both pleased and embarrassed with this feedback.

He shifted the credit to his colleagues. "I hear it quite broadly that our clients are cared for and understood by the staff. They're not used to that. Mostly it's about authentic caring. They're very street savvy and can read a con. They quickly figure out which staff are genuine.

"Or who is an ally. Sometimes a client will come to me and bellyache about what some staffperson said to them. I don't respond, 'Well, that's not right.' I won't be so political. I'll always be neutral. 'Let me check. Let me ask,' I'll say. Then we go together and talk to them. I try to model constructive ways of dealing with conflict. In whatever I do, I'm trying to support and guide their recovery."

* * *

"The irony about being a music therapist in this setting is that I don't make much music myself. When I worked in long-term care, I could play for four or five hours a day. Here I might play piano at a relaxation group, but not always. I also have good recorded music that is as effective. Mostly I'm working with clients on lyrics, or helping them make recordings, and doing a whole lot of talking."

The pace of our conversation had slowed. Antonio had told me plenty about his work, and now he was starting to reflect on what it means to him. It takes time to find the right words to convey emotional undertones to a stranger who is unfamiliar with one's world.

"What about the need to be entrepreneurial, to hustle for jobs, that seems to characterize the careers of so many music therapists?" I prompted.

"My career has consisted entirely of part-time jobs, which has its pros and cons. It's the kind of career where I ask, 'Why the hell did I ever go into this?' while loving it and thinking it makes so much sense. Why didn't I do something more practical? Or at least more portable."

"Portable?"

"It's hard to just up and go. If I wanted to apply at a different hospital, there aren't many openings that come available. I can't just move to, say, Vancouver or Calgary, without serious ramifications. In music therapy, everywhere you go, you have to start over, looking for jobs and pioneering. I'm very much tied to the two jobs I have here, without many options for relocating.

"I could scramble as a freelancer, knitting together numerous small contracts. As I age, though, being full-time is increasingly on my mind, what with benefits and pension considerations. Plus

I'm doing way too much with two jobs. I agree that there's no such thing as two half-time jobs for a salaried employee, only two sixty-percent jobs. Yes, it's absurd, and there's no simple solution.

"Whenever there are increases in staffing and people are getting bumped up into full-time, it seldom feels to me that music therapy is high enough on the priority list, even though the program is really popular and I work throughout the entire centre. Being popular is both good and bad. An occupational therapist will have a caseload of twenty-five. I can carry all seventy people, potentially. That alone would be craziness with part-time hours."

He stared at me. "I have a real love-hate relationship with this career."

I had heard that sentiment before. "Is love-hate typical of the profession?"

"Yes, for sure. I think just about everybody says that." He continued, after a brief break, "Maybe people complain in other professions too, but at least most professions are well established. It's wearing to spend an entire career explaining and pioneering and justifying why your field matters."

We sat in silence, a comfortable silence from my perspective. Finally I raised a topic that had been on mind throughout the conversation, but which we hadn't touched upon. I asked what it was like to be a male in a female-dominated occupation.

I felt awkward as soon as the words came out of my mouth. All my adult life, I've listened and participated in discussions about women in the workplace and, more generally, about the status of women in our society. I was fine with that—supportive, in fact. But to raise the same issues about my gender felt strange and a little gauche. My empathy grew for the many women who, over the decades, decided to initiate uncomfortable, but necessary, conversations concerning gender.

"At this facility," Antonio replied, "the clientele is three-quarters male. Sometimes guys like being with guys when they're doing music. Maybe they feel less need to impress or look competent. Anyhow, there's comfort when it's all male or all female.

"I like having a female partner because some clients are more comfortable with one gender than the other, or with one personality style—it's not only about gender."

Client expectations can be significant and, in some respects, even self-fulfilling. Among the different approaches to providing therapy, some are more permissive or emotion-based. If a client is looking for a therapist who is kinder or softer, their gender stereotypes can kick in and they may look for a female therapist. "I don't think all female therapists are motherly," Antonio said. "Yet, some are. Certain clients respond well to this, so that rewards the therapist for taking a softer approach. It proves effective, so they continue using it."

He continued, "If I'm pushy with clients about working hard and getting at their issues, they can see me as paternalistic—that's how their old man treated them. If a woman therapist does that, then she's seen as a bitch. Clients do have those kinds of reactions.

"Client expectations are deeply embedded. When I'm kind to clients, some of them don't know what to do with that, because they haven't had that experience before.

"I'm not sure whether it's male-female or just my own style, but I'm quite forthright with clients. Sometimes I call it the frying pan technique: when you just have to bonk them on the head about something they need to take more seriously. Not in a mean way, just to help them with their recovery."

Another example of expectations that Antonio said annoyed him is the assumption that males are experts with technology. "When something like an MP3 player is on the blink, clients want me to come and fix it. I have a female colleague who knows this equipment way better than I do, but they just try to mansplain it to her. We chuckle about that."

"Okay, I get how clients have expectations and make assumptions," I said. "What about your colleagues? Does being a man make any difference when you attend conferences or network? Does it affect how you socialize?"

Antonio quickly said it didn't. "The only small rub with colleagues arises more because of my age. I've supervised a number of interns over the years, and sometimes they still see me, just a tiny bit, more as a mentor than a colleague.

"Honestly, the only time I recall the gender card coming up was when somebody questioned why I got this job. 'Because he's male' was the tongue-in-cheek response. I could shrug that off because I knew I was well qualified for the position."

Not much was emerging from what could have been a hot button topic, but then Antonio mentioned a wrinkle I hadn't considered. "Feminism has influenced the various approaches to music therapy, just as it has some other types of therapy. It calls for the removal of hierarchy, as much as possible. In our field, this can mean working co-operatively and sharing. In geriatrics, for example, clients can get all excited when their music therapist gets married. They're happy to participate in the therapist's life, and vice versa. Both male and female therapists can be feminists.

"In some settings, I do share about myself and join in all the activities. But not so much here. In fact, I rarely self-disclose when I work with clients who have concurrent disorders."

I nodded and said something innocuous to encourage him, wondering where he was going with this topic.

An article he had written for a scholarly journal included a case study from his rap program. The peer reviewers criticized him, quite harshly, for not having written and recorded a rap himself, along with clients. "It was reasonable, from a feminist perspective, for them to ask why I had stayed on the sidelines. I wrote back to give my rationale, which partly had to do with my desire not to be a distraction during the limited time available, or to outskill the clients. More significantly, the themes of the raps concerned things I've never experienced firsthand. I can't write something fake, or superficial, and expect my clients to go deep.

"I thought my explanation would be sufficient, even if the reviewers happened to think I hadn't made the best choice. It wasn't. Just the opposite. Now they were really upset, claiming that my efforts to serve my clients were excessively patriarchal. It seemed to me that they were ideologically committed to a certain methodology, whereas I see music therapy as offering a variety of techniques from which to choose, depending on the context."

I asked, "Was it really as big a deal as you're making it sound?"

"I wouldn't have thought so. But, apparently, I was wrong. It still leaves me with a bit of a bad taste. But I remind myself that it was just one incident, which isn't too shoddy, considering all my years in the field. And circling back to your original question about gender, I don't think this had anything to do with me being a man. Though, of course, maybe the problem is that I'm a man, and therefore don't see the problem." He smiled.

He interrupted me as I prepared to speak. "Just one more thing, if I may. It's about self-disclosure."

"Of course."

"Unlike some recovery centres, few staff here have been through addiction themselves. Some of those who have are open about it. Clients love that openness. And even I'll acknowledge a few other types of problems I've faced, without spending much time on them or giving many details, and that's often appreciated. Clients like it when our learning and expertise hasn't come solely from textbooks."

* * *

I proposed we wrap up by talking about the field generally, and how the public perceives it.

"You mean, like people thinking I'm an entertainer or that I do singalongs all day long?" Antonio asked.

"Sure, that seems like a good place to start. How do you cope with those perceptions?"

"I usually give examples of a couple of programs I do, so they can start to see the variety in our practice. But, increasingly, the people I run into, they're getting it right away. They've seen it somewhere or they know somebody, perhaps a friend whose autistic child went to see somebody. So they're realizing the richness.

"In mental health, maybe less so, but people think it makes sense. They maybe don't understand how it looks. Or they've seen a music therapist who practices differently and doesn't have a studio full of equipment and the same resources I'm blessed with here.

"It's interesting how one of the ways our field grows is through practicum placements. On the last practicum, the supervisor doesn't have to be a music therapist. So sometimes students can talk an employer into taking them on for free, for that last practicum, in a place that has never had music therapy before. Employers get to see what a therapist actually does and perhaps say, 'Oh, we want more of this. How do we hire somebody?' That's proven valuable.

"But, but. There's often a catch. The employer wonders how much music therapy is really needed. 'Does it have to be full-time?' We're such a particular niche that we end up on the bottom rung, despite staff in other fields valuing our contribution. We end up having to prove ourselves, yet again.

"As well as among employers, the field itself has inertia and resistance. Some therapists find it hard to get away from the idea that you're supposed to play piano and guitar all day, and nothing else. Well, no. It's okay to use YouTube or recordings. Or make recordings. Or make music electronically. There are so many possibilities, and yet we don't make full use of them.

"Still, lots of niche courses are emerging, like how to apply music therapy in a neonatal intensive care setting or how to use neurologic music therapy for specialized brain training. Almost too many options in an already small profession."

Antonio seemed to have exhausted what he felt I needed to know, so I asked, "What about any tension between therapists who are more oriented towards the humanities and social sciences versus those who are more medical and scientific? Is that a significant issue?"

"Yes, I think they're always a little at odds. Music therapy has long had a feel-good thread, drawing on some hippie origins in the 1960s. It shows up as a qualitative bent in research papers. At the same time, the field values rigour and proof, partly as a way to legitimize and justify our work to other professionals and partly to help us improve the effectiveness of our practice. I gather that other fields, like sociology, also struggle with balancing soft and hard orientations. We're not unique."

"Rigour, but not only rigour?"

"I guess that's a way to describe it." He stroked his chin meditatively while his eyes narrowed, a little mischievously I thought. "Another tension I could talk about is whether music therapy is just to help individuals or whether it should also try to change the system those individuals are in. That involves concepts like building identity, empowerment, and agency. I could tell you about some excellent work on community music therapy coming out of Norway, for example. Would you like a synopsis of Stige and Aarø's 2012 book?"

I regretfully declined a briefing and, after offering profuse thanks, I took my leave. I almost made it out the building, but the doors were locked from both sides. Antonio ambled over and released me. It had been a good session.

MEGAN

The COVID-19 pandemic scuttled my hope of visiting an in-patient rehabilitation unit. Megan, the music therapist, proposed we meet instead in the hospital's education and research wing. "It's largely deserted now that most educational programs have moved online or been suspended, and a lot of people are working from home. There's an outside entrance, so you won't have to cross paths with any patients or staff."

We were comfortably ensconced in vinyl armchairs in the otherwise empty lobby. After making introductions, we commented on some of the inanities brought about by social distancing during the pandemic.

"You know," she said, "sometimes even in normal times, I just have to shake my head. My work has some bizarre aspects."

"How so?"

"Well, one of my Catch-22s is that because music therapy is sort of fun, it isn't taken seriously. Yet, if clients don't like the music and don't get emotionally invested in it, many of my techniques don't work nearly as well."

I must have wrinkled my brow, because she elaborated. "Physiotherapy can be painful and exhausting. Speech work can be tedious. My therapy, in contrast, is rather pleasant, so clients can feel like they're on a break when they see me. I'm tempted at times to inflict on them music that they heartily dislike, just to remind them that we're actually working, but that would be counterproductive. It's positive emotion and engagement that foster the remarkable changes the brain is capable of making with music."

I said this situation sounded like a parent complaining that their child couldn't be learning much because they enjoyed school a great deal. Megan opened her mouth to speak but a concrete drill drowned her words. Evidently pandemic shutdowns are prime times for catching up on deferred maintenance. We retreated outside to an unpainted picnic table on the lawn, hoping our jackets would be adequate, but confident the rain would hold off.

✳ ✳ ✳

"Could you give me some background," I asked, "about your workplace and how you fit in? For example, are you an employee or a self-employed contractor?"

"An employee, part-time. Salaried positions used to be unusual, but being an employee is becoming more common. I gather some hospitals have therapists who get paid through a fundraising foundation and not by a health authority."

"And your unit, what exactly happens there?"

"It's mostly rehabilitation after severe brain and spinal cord injuries. Clients typically come and stay with us for short periods, which in my rehab world means two or three months. That's shorter than it used to be. They have to be showing improvement, and be likely to continue to improve, to get admitted. If a client declines, or even plateaus, it can be heart-wrenching for all of us, especially if they happen to have young children. Then we know the family is going to have a really, really hard life.

"I work mainly with adults, the vast majority as in-patients. The adolescent program has diminished quite a bit. That's a funding issue and reflects management's priorities for our region.

"Sometimes I'm willing to assess patients elsewhere in the hospital and make recommendations, but I really prefer to focus on a specific population. I don't want to be spread so thin as to be seen as the musical entertainer who is just soothing people. I want to work on specific goals. So it's people with strokes and brain injury."

Megan clasped her hands loosely, placing her elbows on the table. I had noticed the purple tinges in her short-cropped dark hair when we met. Now when I raised my eyes from my notepaper, the piercings in her left ear caught my attention. Rather more than usual, but the effect was striking.

I asked where she typically sees clients and how much time she spends with them.

"I have my own office and that's where things usually happen. It's more of a studio, with lots of space for a piano and all sorts of other instruments.

"In order to provide a good exposure to music therapy, I typically see people two or three times a week as opposed to once a week. Usually twice because it's hard for them to slot me into their weekly schedule more than that. A session is generally an hour long. If people have a shorter attention span, I might do half an hour, two or three times a week.

"I almost always work one-on-one because everyone has their own musical preferences and their own specific goals. We could do drumming or playing melodic instruments or listening or singing. All sorts of different things. I may have to track people down, because they forget to come or something else has come up."

"So no groups?" I asked.

"Very few. Before COVID, I ran a Music for Stress Management group. Stress is my code word for "anxiety" because anxiety isn't really a buy-in for a client. Any patient who's in our unit has their sympathetic nervous system in overdrive."

Megan anticipated my question. "That's the system controlling rapid, involuntary responses to dangerous situations. The patient's foot is always on the gas pedal, so to speak. So I'm trying to teach them how to calm everything down. For example, creating a playlist of songs that soothe and relax them. It's a way of involving more people in music therapy."

She smiled, a little impishly I thought, as she added that there's abundant evidence about music stimulating the parasympathetic nervous system. "That's the rest-and-digest system. If nothing else, I want to make sure you leave with lots of medical terminology, Bob."

"Just remember that each time you use it, I'll probably have to ask you how to spell it. Could you tell me what your typical day looks like?"

"That's tough. How about I try describing a typical week? It at least always begins the same way."

"Okay."

"I start by attending rounds, where the professionals update each other about their clients. Progress, problems, if the professional is going to try something new, and so on. I like hearing what's happening in the team and deciding whether I need to chat individually with any of them at a later time. This sharing also helps with scheduling each client's time.

"Rounds can be a little challenging because I don't work with every client. I really have to pipe up if I'm going to say anything because the others aren't expecting to hear from me.

"The purpose of rounds is to talk about barriers to discharge. I'm no barrier. However, what actually happens is that people just give progress reports. Their comments are always goal related, such as fine motor function or providing support for coping and adjustment. It's a very medical model."

I picked up on Megan's use of the word "team." Health educators emphasize the importance of holistic, coordinated care, but the realities of the workplace often push caregivers into parallel silos, where they make valiant but sometimes inadequate efforts to synchronize what they're doing. "Because there's a small group of you working intensely with a small group of clients for a couple of months at a time, do you actually achieve decent teamwork?"

Megan considered my question for a moment. "We do not do too badly, but it's still less than ideal." She proceeded to describe a woman in her twenties who was "bed-seeking," which is the term for somebody who is unmotivated, often due to depression or pain, and tries to dodge their rehabilitation work. "I went into her room and just stood next to her bed, strumming my guitar. She perked her head up and said, 'Hey, you're pretty good.'"

Megan and I laughed at this. "Clients sometimes just say what's on their mind. They don't always have a filter after their injury, which can be very refreshing. Anyhow, I was able to persuade her to do some music therapy. Then I said, 'Since you're up, what do you think about going down to physio now?' I got her up, she'd come for music, and then others took her somewhere else. That's a type of teamwork."

Returning to the topic of rounds, Megan said that she and a recreation therapist have sometimes complained that the medical model leaves them feeling discounted. Yet they have fresh perspectives to bring to the table. "It's not unusual for somebody to report that John Doe isn't very motivated and to see most of the other professionals around the table nodding in agreement. I might say he shows up regularly with me and is very engaged. Maybe, I tactfully suggest, the problem is us, not him. Maybe the problem is the emotional environment we're creating for him.

"The role of the emotions in healing, especially joy, tends to get slighted in the push to help the client with their physical recovery. I remember one client who was becoming overwhelmed by the intensity of a busy schedule. The person making the report concluded, 'So we'll drop music and rec therapy entirely for the next week or two.' This really annoyed me because that approach wasn't client centred. There were lots of goals for that client, many of which could also be addressed through music and rec therapy. This situation provided a great opportunity for physio, occupational, and speech therapies to really liaise with us in providing results-oriented sessions for our client. But, unfortunately, no one else saw it that way, except music and rec therapy."

Megan then seemed to remember that she had embarked on describing a typical week. "The rest of the week is just seeing various clients."

I waited for her to elaborate but she remained silent. I wondered if she was thinking about other examples of feeling undervalued that she didn't want to share with me. Finally I asked, "What about charting? How much of a burden is that?

She tilted her head back, looking at the sky as she grinned and gently rolled her head from side to side. "And charting. Yes, I do some charting." She sighed. "Scheduling is so challenging, because people are fully booked. I'm trying to squeeze in a little time here, and a little there, with each of my clients. So I kind of chart whenever I can, but client appointments take priority. Sometimes I fall a couple of weeks behind. I have a music therapy assessment that I should do and put in the chart. Sometimes that doesn't happen. But I usually go to rounds and speak up when I'm involved in the person's care.

"Our charting is interdisciplinary. I could write directly under a doctor's note. Or nursing. We're all writing in the progress notes, so everybody sees what everyone else is saying. If, that is, they read all the notes added since the last time they looked at the chart. There's nothing online yet. It's paper charting.

"I hear that at some other places, charts have different sections for each profession. Unless a reader looks in the right section, they're not going to know about music therapy."

Megan examined me, as if she searching for clues about whether her description of the process had satisfied me. I asked about her role in discharge planning.

"Sometimes I add recommendations to the discharge summary. I might, for example, recommend ongoing access or exposure to music. A real problem is that sometimes there aren't enough music therapists in the community to allow me to recommend actual music therapy. Many people can't afford a private therapist, especially if they face hefty costs for the rest of their lives to purchase disability supports and supplies. It's a funding issue and can be hard to solve. I don't want to recommend music therapy if people are likely going to find they can't afford it when they look into it."

She added that funding is occasionally available from insurance companies, such as after a car accident. "They might fund music therapy, but only if the person has played music in the past, which is really beside the point. This approach shows a lack of understanding of music therapy and all its applications."

Something about the topic of discharge planning took Megan full circle, because she started talking about her first session with a client. "It's always what I call a meet and greet. I ask them what sorts of things they're working on and I explain how music might be able to help. Then I leave music therapy as a choice. If they want to come back, I tell them they don't have to sing if they don't want to. That's a common concern."

"Any final comments about your workplace before we move on?" I asked.

"No, not really. For the most part, I thoroughly enjoy working here. Every client is different. I like the flexibility and creativity of the job."

* * *

Megan grew up in a musical family. She trained classically on the piano and sang in choirs, at church and elsewhere. She completed a music degree in the eastern United States, with the intention of returning to Canada to take additional training to become a schoolteacher.

During her music studies, the university awarded her a bursary, one which required her to volunteer somewhere in the community—a nice relationship the university had developed with the city and a résumé-builder for the student. She chose to volunteer at an elementary school, only to find the school system's structure and lack of flexibility put her off. "I also learned that their music teachers often have to work at more than one school, meaning they have to pack things in the trunk of their car and drive. So I wasn't sure that was for me.

"Then I volunteered with a woman who offered a music group for little kids, many of whom had diverse abilities. I loved it. I thought it was really cool how a preschooler could light up and come out of themselves just through music. I became interested in music as a tool for helping people."

Now quite uncertain what she wanted to do with her life, Megan took a gap year and travelled to Australia, working in jobs that had nothing to do with either music or education. She remained unsure upon returning to Canada. What nudged her to finally make a decision was that during Megan's time abroad, her aunt had suffered a stroke. "This helped me become familiar and comfortable with people with disabilities. Visiting her in long-term care, I could see how music made the residents' faces brighten. That experience reinforced the different understanding of music I had gained as a volunteer in university.

"I decided to look into this music therapy thing. I didn't know if I would pursue it, but I thought I'd give myself permission to study it and see what happened. That was fourteen years ago."

Megan considered two places to study music therapy. One, in Ontario, required her to do a qualifying year before she could apply for admission. "That didn't appeal to me. I'd always wanted to live out west, to see what it's like, so I ended up North Vancouver. I had to pick up a course in biology and another in psychology, but then I went straight into third year at Capilano."

I was curious about the extent to which her time at Capilano University had changed her as a musician, quite apart from the therapeutic focus of her studies. She explained that she acquired a wider range of styles, since people have a broad span of musical tastes and therapists have to be prepared to work with any of them. "The big thing, though, was learning how to improvise. This was completely foreign to me as a classical piano player, as someone who performs pieces exactly as written. That was a big learning curve, but very freeing. Then you're appreciating the process of making music as opposed to the end product. I also learned another instrument, the guitar. I was even playing piano differently."

"How did you come to get a job in a rehab unit?" I asked. "Was this something that interested you during your studies or did it happen after you were fully qualified?"

As is so often the case, it turned out that a work placement during her studies had put her on this path. "My friend had done her last practicum on the unit, once a week. Her stories interested me. When my supervisor suggested rehab as one of my internship sites, partly because she had a friend there who could be my onsite mentor, I immediately agreed. My other internship site was at another place with little kids.

"My fascination grew with how music affects the brain. I just loved it. The interdisciplinary aspect also appealed to me. I could chat with the speech language pathologists, learning what they're doing. Also the occupational therapists, physiotherapists, recreation therapists, social workers. It was really great.

"And my timing was good. The hospital had recently realized the benefits of music therapy, and a couple of programs agreed to reallocate some of their budget to create a music therapy position. I will be forever grateful. It took a number of months, and I had to apply and compete for the job, but I was lucky enough to get the position."

"And you've been there ever since?"

"Yes. It's a good fit."

I had seen on Megan's website that she also has a counselling degree, one that I deduced she must have obtained after becoming a music therapist. "Did you see your counselling studies as an extension of the therapy work you were already doing or more as a change of pace?"

"Definitely an extension. Though I did think it would be nice to do a little straight counselling, just for variety."

Megan explained that she encounters a lot of regret and grief in people with major head and spinal cord injuries. She wanted more counselling skills in order to support them better. "When people come in, their life has changed dramatically. Their life has transformed in a second and that's it. Even with slow-growing brain tumours, there's a sudden change when they receive the diagnosis. There might be some damage from the surgery. Clients talk about their life as the times before and after the accident, before and after the injury.

"They had hopes and dreams, and those hopes are often dashed. Sometimes their partners leave. They're fretting about what's next. There's a lot of grief, and sometimes guilt. Don't ever underestimate the long-term psychological impact of a chronic illness or a profound injury."

I fully appreciated the importance of Megan's comments, but I wanted to cover a couple of other topics in our limited time together. I observed that she was certainly well educated.

"Yes," she said. "Maybe I got a little carried away. I did a Bachelor of Music, then a Bachelor of Music Therapy, and a Master's in Counselling Psych. Now I'm doing this advanced training in the Bonny Method of Guided Imagery and Music, and that's almost like another master's. So I have as much or more education than the doctors I work with."

"Too bad you don't get paid anywhere near the same as them," I quipped. She agreed.

"Story time," I announced. "It's time for you to tell me about some of your cases, if that's the right word. And I wouldn't grumble if you started with something on the more dramatic end of the scale."

Megan scowled. "You're sounding a little demanding and directive, don't you think?"

"Yes," I readily agreed. "And I'm going to pout until I get what I want." I leaned back and folded my arms.

"Nice try, but you're a teddy bear compared to some of the clients I see. Let me tell you about one of them, a teenager who I'll call Allen."

Allen's prospects for playing professional baseball had been very good. Scouts from across the USA had started calling him, urging him to consider their organization when he graduated from high school in half a year's time. Then came a frosty patch of road and a devastating car crash. He eventually surfaced in Megan's rehab unit.

"When you're super athletic and young, you tend to recover well physically. He could walk normally in almost no time at all. But his brain was damaged, and he didn't really remember where he was or understand what was happening to him. He became increasingly frustrated, punching the wall and generally acting out. His doc was fabulous and pretty clued in about music therapy. He asked me if I could have a go at working with Allen to help with anger management."

Allen arrived on time at Megan's door, a security guard in tow because he was prone to violence. She introduced herself and said, "I do music around here. Are you interested in any music?"

Allen swore at her, and then added that he wasn't interested, just in case she'd missed the point.

"Okay," Megan replied evenly. "But I have 2Pac in my office, if you ever change your mind."

"You have 2Pac!" Allen exclaimed and stepped into her office.

"Two what?" I asked. I'm not very up on pop culture.

"Tupac Shakur," Megan told me. "He's a rapper who was killed in a gang war. There are some amazing theories that he may have faked his own death or somehow still be alive. He's like a modern-day Elvis. I get a bit of street credibility when I can join the speculation as to whether he's really dead."

Megan resumed her story. "I put on the CD, and he immediately starts bouncing and swaying. Before long, he's dancing to it. Then he persuades the security guard to join in, so I follow suit. All three of us are dancing to 2Pac, and I'm trying to prolong it until I figure out what on earth I'm going to do next. Eventually an idea comes to me.

"'Do you hear that drum?' I asked him. 'The beat in that song? I bet you could do that.' I have a drum set in my office, so now he's playing the drums. This is a strategy to get him engaged in all kinds of thinking, cognitive skills. I'd show him a pattern, very basic. Then he could do whatever he wanted, going to town on the drums. That's getting out frustrations, a physical outlet. Then I'd say, 'Oh, what's the pattern again?' Back and forth, working on short-term memory.

"He had a blast. It was fabulous. He was a great kid, lots of fun to work with. And being a competitive guy, I could show him a pattern on the drums and say, 'I'm going to try to distract you by playing something else. I'm going to try to mess up what you're doing.' His challenge was to stay with his rhythm pattern and not get distracted by me. That's all about focus and concentration. There were lots of ways I was able to use music to help him.

"Next, I put him on the electric bass. All you need to know is four strings. So I got some music, the theme from the TV show *Friends*—even though it's dated, he really liked the show. He just had to read second string, third string, and so on. That's how I wrote it out, without the proper string names, so that he could play. He had to look at the music, then the strings, then look back at the music and know where he was on the page. There's a lot of skills for him to work on, plus he's now a bass player. He's feeling pretty cool and really enjoying himself.

"His mom sat in for one of the sessions and was thrilled. This was probably the first time she'd felt any hope of getting her son back, rather than a body that looked like her son.

"I often don't know what happens after people leave us. Our work is just a small part of the overall recovery. But I do know that when this guy went back to his community, supports were in place so that he could continue to play music. He could play with people of a similar ability, under the leadership of a music therapist. I had helped him find a new outlet and experience the thrill of acquiring a new skill. There was no way he could go back to his old sport, but now he had a glimpse of a different life that he could build for himself."

We sat in comfortable silence for a moment, savouring the story. "So you give your clients the option of singing or not, but it seems like dancing is compulsory?" I asked.

"Only if they're mobile. And hip."

I became more serious. "Allen sounds like he was one of your memorable, special clients." Megan nodded in agreement. "Could you give me a couple of examples of the more typical clients, perhaps people you've worked with recently."

Megan said "typical" is a word they rarely get to use on her unit, but she knew what I meant. "I encounter such a range of people. Yesterday, for example, I had somebody whose only musical interest is Chinese opera. I, of course, don't know any, nor could I possibly learn to sing those high pitches—it's just out of my league. But we could listen to recordings. My carefully chosen questions, asking what was going on in the various scenes, helped him with his cognitive goals.

"Coincidentally, I recently finished with another client who, like Allen, also started out full of anger. He had overdosed on quite a few drugs. While he was fine cognitively, he had damaged himself physically. The worst was losing his sight.

"Tomoya was extremely frustrated, and our staff had a hard time managing his outbursts and refusals to co-operate. Eventually the powers that be concluded they'd have to transfer him elsewhere. While that decision was being made, I happened to have helped him write a song, a process that required plenty of patience because he also had a speech problem. The lyrics revealed someone who was really scared and needed people in his life. It enabled staff to see him in a whole new way, coming to understand that his behaviour was really his grief expressing itself. He stayed with us for another month, leaving just a week or two ago."

We waited while a garbage truck lifted a dumpster over its cab and emptied the contents, giving it a couple of extra shakes for good measure. The loading bay amplified the clanging of metal on metal, causing a pedestrian in the driveway to grimace. Two crows circled briefly overhead, then perched in an ornamental maple near our table.

"Sometimes I have people who have had a stroke and can't talk," Megan said, "but they can sing because it comes from a different part of the brain. It's rather amazing. Let me think of a case to tell you about." She rested her cheek on her hand and resumed talking.

"Martina had an aneurism in her twenties. When she first came to me, she could only say a single word at a time, not even a phrase, but she could sing long passages. Fortunately, she loved singing and knew all sorts of songs. We'd do entire songs from the Backstreet Boys, even rounds, and everything sounded smooth upon a casual hearing. If you listened closely, though, you'd detect a lost syllable or two, or the wrong syllable. That's a motor planning problem, called apraxia."

Megan spelled the word for me and explained that it can manifest in several ways. "The brain knows what it wants to say but can't properly plan and sequence the required speech sound movements. It just doesn't quite work. You might reach out for something but go too far. Apraxia affects intended movement of arms and legs, as well as speech.

"I wasn't at all surprised to learn that Martina was working on syllables in Speech. They'd do a beat for each syllable to even out her speech and make sure nothing got lost. It's easy to trip up over multisyllabic words. There's a lot we take for granted when we speak, and it's the slowest ability to return.

"Reinforcing what she was doing in Speech was right up my alley. When, for example, we did the song "Hallelujah," I'd set up drums so she'd have to hit them and get the timing.

"She was fond of a Justin Bieber tune. I'm not a fan of his, though at least I don't suffer as much with him as with Britney Spears. But I suck it up for my clients, if that's what they like. Anyway, in the middle of this Bieber song, there's an instrumental solo. I pulled out a xylophone for her to play the solo. That's working on her eye-hand coordination, with motor planning. The passage was a bit challenging, which is good. I wanted to push her but not overwhelm her.

"She was very motivated in all her rehab and it was fun working with her. As she progressed, her goals became more complex. Gradually she came to say what she wanted to work on during a session, rather than me always directing her.

"By way of an example, she told me one day that she wanted to practise enunciation, a component of her oral-motor goals. If I recall correctly, one of the songs we used was the *Sesame Street* song "Mah Nà Mah Nà." We did it slowly, emphasizing the 'em' and 'en' sounds. We also worked a bit on gait, because when you're walking to music, the movement is easier and more efficient due to the way it's processed in the brain.

"Reading and recognizing words were a challenge for her. I printed out the days of the week and taped them randomly to a music stand. There's a Sting piece where he's singing the days of the week. She would point to the day and sing it with me when I sang it. This was just another way of supporting her existing goals.

"She was a rewarding client to work with. At the beginning, as I mentioned, she could say little more than a single syllable. After about half a year, seeing me twice a week and working with a speech language pathologist, she was able to tell me she needed more practice in recognizing the days of the week. Then I got to see her as an outpatient once a week for another eight or nine months."

Not every day, but often enough, Megan has to support clients struggling with profound emotions. Sometimes, for example, sad and terrible things happen during childbirth, such as a stroke or insufficient oxygen reaching a mother's brain. Once she's medically stable, the new mother may receive rehabilitation as an inpatient. "She wants to get back to her baby as soon as possible, not work on her own recovery. So what can I do for her in music therapy? I usually suggest we learn some songs for her to sing to her baby, and it can do wonders. I can subtly address any cognitive goals for the mother. More importantly, this strategy partially normalizes a situation that is anything but normal. It helps to affirm the mother as a caregiver and parent, while giving her a few tools to soothe and bond with her baby when they do eventually reunite."

I misinterpreted Megan's glance at her watch. "I could listen all day," I said, "but perhaps just one more story." She raised her eyebrows and shrugged in agreement.

"You may have gathered," she said, "that I really like the interdisciplinary approach. Sometimes we accomplish more together than we could individually. Here's an example of what I mean, although once again it was me initiating the collaboration. No matter how many presentations they hear, it's still mainly my personal one-on-ones with other professionals that keep my interdisciplinary work alive.

"'Hey,' I said to a physiotherapist, 'we're both working with Jane. My hunch is that she'd progress faster with both of us present for a few of her sessions.' Long story cut short: when Jane went home, she only needed a walking stick and not a walker. That may sound minor, but not all bathroom doorways can handle the width of a walker. Sometimes it's tough to find space to swing the walker around and position it so that you can sit safely on the toilet. And every time you get in or out of bed, you need room to manoeuvre the walker around bedside tables and dressers. Having to deal with just a cane makes a huge difference.

"Everybody was pleased. The physio said in rounds how much music had helped Jane regain mobility, boosting her to the next level. That really made my day, though of course we professionals continued to fall back into our familiar silos and not work together as much as we desire."

✸ ✸ ✸

This last story struck me as a good opportunity to segue into a topic I wanted to explore thoroughly. "I'm sure people in all sorts of organizations," I said as blandly as possible, "get frustrated trying to promote teamwork when there are so many pressures pushing us back into our occupational boxes. Every workplace has its challenges, no matter how good it is. I'm wondering what sorts of challenges you regularly face, because the books and videos I've seen have emphasized the good side of music therapy. The spins are all positive. The things that bug you might not be big or serious, but knowing about them would help me get a more realistic picture of your world."

I held my breath as Megan pondered my request. I wondered if she would be comfortable with this line of questioning or whether she would shut it down. Finally she replied, "The perpetual challenge for all of us in this field is that people don't fully understand what we do." She flicked her hands up and outwards. "The hardest are the people who think they absolutely know what music therapy is, but they're wrong. The ones who know they're clueless, at least you can have teachable moments with them.

"Recently a client told me her relative is a music therapist. Something seemed dubious about this claim, so I casually asked where she had trained. 'Oh, she didn't train anywhere.' It was the same when I chatted with the relative, 'Oh no, I just do it.' Psychologists and some other professionals face this sort of naivety, so I'm not alone. But it can be frustrating when people are oblivious to the skills and knowledge needed to do any sort of therapy well."

"Does anything that extreme ever happen with your co-workers?" I asked. "The know-it-alls, I mean."

Megan shook her head. "No, thank goodness. The problem on my unit is more a lack of knowledge about music therapy, not incorrect knowledge. I join with a few others who are one-of-a-kind in rehab in an annual or semi-annual education event for our colleagues. We take turns talking about what we do, giving clinical examples, and identifying good areas for collaboration. The audience consists mainly of people who want to learn about our fields and who would probably eventually figure it out in any event. It's harder to reach the others who don't attend.

"I suppose one of my bigger bugbears related to people's lack of knowledge about music therapy is getting typecast. In some people's view, all I'm capable of doing is playing music for patients. That's it. As much as I describe how music therapy can provide emotional support for somebody who is struggling with depression, or even temporarily feeling low, when this topic comes up in rounds, everyone turns to the psychologist or social worker. I get a little tired of saying, 'Hey, perhaps I have something to offer.' The constant need for me to advocate about my skill set, and remind others that I can help with emotions, can be discouraging.

"A while ago, we were short a psychologist. I went to the client's doctor and said that I was a registered clinical counsellor with a master's in counselling psych, so I could see the client, if necessary. She just kind of looked surprised. You get typecast as a musician. People don't see how broad our skills are, or how they transfer to other areas."

I looked up from my clipboard and caught Megan's eye. "I think I may already know the answer to my next question, because it's rampant in health care. But let me ask it anyway. It's the problem of hierarchy, with some doctors and some managers having far too much ego and acting as if they are gods. To what extent is this part of your reality?"

She replied that she didn't experience anything out of the ordinary. "People are mostly good. Probably the worst that happens is that some clinician will decide they need to see the client, and the client's appointment with me simply gets cancelled without consulting me. This doesn't happen often, especially as I make my displeasure known when it does occur."

Most expressions of hierarchy and self-importance in Megan's environment seemed to be subtle rather than flagrant. She described a situation from years ago, when she was fairly new. "One of my clients was having flashbacks to her injury. This concerned me because the injury wasn't due to an accident. She had been deliberately and violently assaulted. I tracked down her doctor in the hallway to have a quick word with him about the case. He snapped at me, asking what made me think I could talk to him right now? I got the feeling he wouldn't have responded in that tone if I had been a physiotherapist. When people behave unprofessionally, it makes you leery of approaching them again with any concerns about clients. It makes you go looking instead for other team members to talk with. That's not good."

I thought about hierarchy for a while but decided not to pursue it further. Instead, I picked up on Megan's comment about being one-of-a kind—the only person on her team offering music therapy. For much of my career, my work situation was similarly unique and I was curious about how her experience might compare to mine. "What's it like for you, being on your own?" I asked.

"Yes, I'm very much alone in a number of respects and have to figure out a lot by myself. The isolation can be a little challenging.

"I can think of one hospital in the province where there actually is a music therapy practice leader, but most of us don't have one. If we do have a leader, it certainly isn't a music therapist. Many of us are linked up with recreation therapy or occupational therapy. Any education or meetings are usually along those bents. Looking back, if I'd had more of a mentor, perhaps there were other things I could have taken advantage of.

"The other complication is that my practice is quite specific, and differs from what many other music therapists do. So even connecting with my peers isn't quite what I would like it to be.

"However, I can fly under the radar. Upper management is aware of me, but they don't know a lot about me. And when it comes to budget-cutting, I'm really not enough to save a lot of money if they get rid of me."

This last statement confused me a little. "Are you saying that the executive group is reluctant to cut music therapy because it can't anticipate the consequences, and in any event a cut wouldn't save much money?"

"Yes, although I don't know that for sure. That's just how it seems to me. The managers not knowing a lot about what I do is not always an advantage. There's no one really pushing for increased hours in music therapy, unless it's a rather savvy manager. If I say it would be great if I had more hours, they think,

'Well, yeah, of course she's going to say that.' Somebody else needs to advocate for me. But there is no one else. The people we report to are generally not music therapists. They are going to want more hours for their own profession because they can predict exactly what the benefits will be.

Megan shrugged her shoulders. "I don't think about these topics very much. I prefer to focus on clinical work with patients. The admin and political stuff takes a lot of time. I put it to the side as much as I can."

As our conversation lulled, I thought we had reached the end of workplace challenges, but Megan surprised me. "Another thing is evidence-based practice." She searched for another word. "Research." Pause. "Not in the lab or at university. Actual research in clinical settings.

"Getting resources to do research is very political. A number of the grants in health care come from pharmaceutical companies, and why would they fund research into music therapy if it might result in people needing fewer drugs?

"My thing is that music drives neural plasticity. Using a hammer and playing a xylophone involve pretty much the same arm movements and eye-hand coordination, but you're using more of your brain with the xylophone. So it makes sense to use music in rehabilitation. We need as much documented evidence as possible to drive this point home.

"Research about music and the brain can be complicated because it's very important that the subjects like the music they're hearing. If every subject in an experiment likes something a little different, then it becomes hard to find a matching control group to measure the impact of, say, the frequency and duration of a therapy.

"Another challenge is differentiating between short- and long-term effects. When I was in my counselling psychology program,

I read a fair amount about cognitively based behavioural therapies. I wasn't a fan of the research because a lot of the outcomes were measured just two or four months later. It was short term. Sometimes people need long-term stuff for complicated grief.

"Anyhow, coming back to my situation, I was able to conduct some research about pain and mood among my clients. I presented the findings around the hospital, and my audiences thought that it was a good study. But health care is so overworked, with so much resulting tunnel vision, that nothing much came of it."

※ ※ ※

At this point, I strongly suspected Megan had given me all the time she could afford. I asked if she had any final observations as we wrapped up.

A shadow passed over her face, ripening into a frown, and then into an expression of considerable discomfort. "I've done what I always do when explaining music therapy. I've talked about the functionality of music, about its ability to address rehab goals, and skipped the part about its aesthetic beauty when dealing with a serious health challenge. I go back and forth between using music as a tool and just pausing with clients to soak in all the beauty."

She explained, "I remember one client for whom regaining some speech was an obvious goal, but he only wanted to listen to music. Nothing else."

"That seems odd," I commented. "Do you know why? Was he afraid of failing or the amount of work involved?"

"It seemed more important to him just to absorb the beauty of music. So I chose to sing a couple of songs that I knew he liked, strumming along on my guitar. He placed his hand over his heart and slowly nodded his head, as if to say, 'Man, I love that song.'

"He struck me as a lonely middle-aged man with little to no social network. Before his devastating stroke, he might have been that quiet guy in the bar who is there for the band, a nice guy who sits at the back and doesn't bother anyone. I tried to work on some cognitive goals by encouraging him to choose songs with the abilities he had, and he did that. Occasionally he would utter a word, and from that I could piece together a bit of how he knew a song. In this way, there was some reminiscence for him, as well as a quality of life. And perhaps a sense of normalcy for him, depending on what he'd done before his injury.

"Experiencing music with someone, as opposed to listening alone, can be very meaningful. What he often needed, trapped in rehab and grieving his old life, was something important to him, not utilitarian. We all need moments that are life-giving and affirm us as human beings."

I mentioned that my neighbours had just had twins. "They desperately need to take an occasional break and simply breathe. The mom, especially, seems so frazzled with the babies that I'm sure she has lost sight of why she wanted kids in the first place."

Megan said that an *aha* moment arrived one June in Colorado during some neurologic training. She had spent the day immersed in terminology and theory about music and the brain. Needing to clear her head, she took a stroll in the evening and happened upon a string quartet playing in a plaza. "The music was so lovely. It made my soul ache. That's when I really came to appreciate the aesthetic beauty of the music itself for weary people. What I had been studying all day was certainly worthwhile, but it utterly failed to take beauty and the human spirit into account."

She went on to describe a stroke victim who had lost so much arm movement that he would never again be able to play his viola. "He indicated a favourite string concerto he used to play, and we listened to it together, letting the sound fill the room. He cried and cried for his loss and the magnitude of his injury. My role was to hold the space so that he could express his grief about a huge loss on his own terms. His speech had been affected, so he couldn't really talk through his feelings with anyone. Perhaps my office was the only safe and available place for him to grieve in this particular way."

After giving me a moment to sit with this story, she continued, "As an aside, highly skilled musicians are not the best candidates for music therapy. We know exactly the sound we're seeking and get distracted while pursuing it. Often I avoid the musician's primary instrument and try to use something entirely different with them."

I said, "I hadn't considered the implications of offering music therapy to a musician. That's interesting."

"Another twist is that I've had some musicians, and even other clients who adore music, refuse to continue with my therapy because it stirs up too much grief in them. I understand. I'd probably be a terrible music therapy client myself."

Megan again glanced at her watch. "Yikes, I'm afraid I have to run. Fortunately, I think that's all I wanted to say. Just email me if you want clarification or have more questions."

As she swung her leg over the bench of the picnic table, she pointed her forefinger at me and urged, "When you write this up, make sure you emphasize the beauty of music and that the ultimate goal of rehab is the quality of the client's life. These don't always make it onto the charts in our medical model of health care." She waved to me over her shoulder as she raced along the sidewalk.

Her parting words stayed with me long after I had pocketed my pen, gathered my notes, and begun making my way home. They struck me as the right note on which to end.

REFERENCES

Online Glimpses

YouTube videos

"How Music Therapy Changed My Life," posted by Children's Hospital Colorado

"An Adult with Autism Shines in Music Therapy," posted by Ryan Judd

"Music Therapy & Emotions for Depression, Stress & Mental Health Issues," posted by Hope E. Young

"Music Therapy Helps People Struggling with Substance Abuse," posted by WIVB TV

"Parkinson's and Music Therapy," posted by Norton Healthcare

"Trauma and Music Therapy: Let the Healing Begin," a TEDx talk by Karla Hawley

"Using Music Therapy to Treat Trauma," posted by Kelly Meashey

Neuroscience

Levitin, D. (2008). *The World in Six Songs: How the Musical Brain Created Human Nature.* New York: Dutton.

Levitin, D. (2006). *This is Your Brain on Music: The Science of a Human Obsession.* New York: Dutton.

Sacks, O. (2007). *Musicophilia: Tales of Music and the Brain.* New York: Alfred A. Knopf.

YouTube videos

"Why I Want to Change the World with Music Therapy," TedxUSFSP talk by Erin Seibert

"Power of Music on the Brain: Dementia and Parkinson's," posted by ABC Science

"Your Brain On Music," TedxPerth talk by Alan Harvey

Becoming a Therapist

YouTube videos

"My Journey to Music Therapy: Becoming an MT-BC," posted by RubatoMT

"My Internship Experience: Becoming a Music Therapist," posted by RubatoMT

Annette

Beitel/Lazar Productions Inc. (Producer). (1999). *On Wings of Song* [DVD]. Montreal.

Stewart, K., Loewy, J., et al. (2005). "The Role of Music Therapy in Care for the Caregivers of the Terminally Ill." In Dileo, Cheryl & Loewy, Joanne (Eds.), *Music Therapy at the End of Life* (pp. 239–250). Cherry Hill, NJ: Jeffrey Books.

Thaut, M., McIntosh, G., & Hoemberg, V. (2014). "Neurologic Music Therapy: From Social Science to Neuroscience." In Thaut, M. & Hoemberg, V. (Eds.). *Handbook of Neurologic Music Therapy* (pp. 1–6). Oxford, UK: Oxford University Press.

Lightning Source UK Ltd.
Milton Keynes UK
UKHW012235021121
393274UK00002B/28